The Cleveland Clinic Guide to

LUNG
CANCER

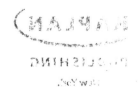

The Cleveland Clinic Guide to

LUNG CANCER

Peter Mazzone, MD

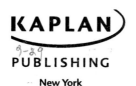

PUBLISHING

New York

This publication is designed to provide accurate and authoritative information in regard to the subject matter covered. It is sold with the understanding that the publisher is not engaged in rendering medical, legal, or other professional service. If medical advice or other expert assistance is required, the services of a competent professional should be sought.

Artwork is reprinted with the permission of The Cleveland Clinic Center for Medical Art & Photograph © 2010.

Published by Kaplan Publishing, a division of Kaplan, Inc.
1 Liberty Plaza, 24th Floor
New York, NY 10006

Printed in the United States of America

10 9 8 7 6 5 4 3 2 1

Library of Congress Cataloging-in-Publication Data

Mazzone, Peter.
    The Cleveland Clinic guide to lung cancer / Peter Mazzone.
    p. cm. — (Cleveland Clinic guide series)
    Includes bibliographical references and index.
    ISBN 978-1-60714-430-4 (alk. paper)
    1. Lungs—Cancer—Popular works. I. Title.
    RC280.L8M32 2010
    616.99'424—dc22

2009028834

Kaplan Publishing books are available at special quantity discounts to use for sales promotions, employee premiums, or educational purposes. Please call the Simon & Schuster special sales department at 866-506-1949.

For my wife Kim,
my daughter Maela,
my parents,
and my family.

Thank you for making my
work and life worthwhile.

Contents

Contents

Introduction

I f you (or someone you care about) have been told that you have or might have lung cancer, you are likely to experience an array of emotions. Most people have a friend or family member who did poorly with a similar diagnosis; thus, hope is not the first emotion that they feel. Many also feel guilt, blaming themselves for lifestyle choices that may have contributed to their health concerns. Often, the deluge of information about the evaluation and treatment of their disease, provided by doctors, well-intentioned family and friends, or the Internet, adds confusion to the mix. In this book, I intend to provide you and your loved ones with a broad overview of the evaluation and management of lung cancer. In so doing, I hope that you'll begin to feel more empowered than guilty, more informed than confused, and more hopeful than fearful.

The early portion of this book will provide you with information about the nature of lung cancer, the testing that may be performed to help diagnose lung cancer, and the means available for your doctors to determine how advanced the cancer is. The goal of these chapters is that you'll become informed enough to participate actively in discussions and decisions about your care. This will help you to be more comfortable with the plans that are made.

The middle of the book will describe the treatments that are available for people with lung cancer. These chapters broadly outline the types of standard treatment for lung cancer of different types and stages. They also provide you with guidance about how to manage the side effects of lung cancer treatment. Each person is unique, so the descriptions given in these chapters can only be considered guidelines. Ultimately, I hope that this information will enable you to have candid discussions with your doctors about the risks and benefits of the treatments that are being suggested to you.

The book ends with chapters intended to provide you with hope and comfort. The chapters describing advances in the evaluation and treatment of lung cancer are the most exciting to me. I hope it leaves you as optimistic as I am about the progress that is being made. The final chapter discusses the possible complications from advanced stages of lung cancer and its treatment. The intention of this chapter is to assure you that people with lung cancer can remain dignified and empowered regardless of the outcome of their illness.

I recognize the challenges that people and their loved ones who are being evaluated or treated for lung cancer face. I hope that the content of this book provides you with enough knowledge and hope to navigate the challenges more easily.

Peter Mazzone, MD, MPH, FRCPC, FCCP
Director of the Lung Cancer Program
Cleveland Clinic Respiratory Institute
www.clevelandclinic.org/pulmonary

Chapter 1

Understanding Lung Cancer

Every time you take a breath—some 10 to 20 times a minute—you inhale air into your lungs, the two spongy, saclike organs in your chest. Protected within a bony cage of 12 sets of ribs, your lungs are among the largest organs in your body. When you breathe in, your lungs expand with air, and oxygen is absorbed into your bloodstream. As you breathe out, your lungs deflate and push out carbon dioxide, the waste gas produced as part of your metabolism. Just beneath your lungs is your diaphragm, a dome-shaped sheet of muscle that moves your lungs each time you inhale and exhale.

Breathing begins when you inhale air through your nose or mouth. The air travels down your throat and into your trachea (windpipe). As your trachea joins your lungs, it divides at a point called the main carina into two airways, called bronchi, that lead into either lung. Each bronchus (the singular of bronchi) then divides, like the branches of a tree, into many thousands of smaller and smaller airways called bronchioles. The smallest bronchioles connect to tiny air-filled sacs called alveoli. The average adult's lungs contain about 600 million alveoli. Tiny blood vessels called capillaries surround the alveoli. The capillaries and alveoli are where the real work of respiration takes place. Oxygen passes through the thin walls of the alveoli into the capillaries and is carried from there to the rest of your body. Carbon dioxide passes from the capillaries into the alveoli; exhaling carries the carbon dioxide out of your body.

To make room for all those millions of alveoli, your lungs are divided into sections called lobes. Your right lung has three lobes; your left lung has only two lobes and is a little smaller because your heart takes up more room on that side of your body. A thin tissue called the pleura covers your lungs and lines the inside of your chest to protect and cushion the lungs. Between the two layers of the pleura is a very small amount of fluid called the pleural fluid. The pleural fluid lubricates the layers and lets your lungs move smoothly when you breathe.

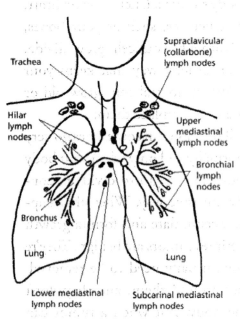

Normal Lung Anatomy

The space in your chest in between your lungs is called the mediastinum; your heart fits snugly there. Wrapped around the trachea and the bronchi are lymph nodes. These small, bean-shaped structures collect lymph, the clear fluid that bathes all the cells in your body and carries nutrients into the cells and waste products away. The white blood cells that are your body's immune system defenders are also found in your lymph nodes. In your chest, chains of lymph nodes lie along the bronchi, along your trachea, and in the mediastinum.

Lung Cancer

The building blocks of your body are cells, the microscopic structures that make up all the tissues of your body. Your cells specialize to become your body's organs (such as your heart, lungs, or brain) and other structures, such as your bones, nerves, muscles, and blood. Normally, your cells grow, divide, and produce more cells in an orderly way that keeps your body functioning properly. When normal cells grow old or are damaged, they die and new cells replace them.

The normal process of cell division can sometimes go very wrong. Instead of dividing normally and only when your body needs them to, cells can sometimes begin to divide uncontrollably and in a disorderly, invasive way. When that happens, the abnormal cells can accumulate and form a growth or mass called a tumor. Sometimes tumors are benign. They're not a threat to life, they don't usually need to be removed, they don't invade the tissues around them, and they don't spread to other parts of the body. But when a tumor can invade nearby tissues and organs, can spread to other parts of the body, and may grow back after being removed, it's malignant—another way of saying cancer.

Lung cancer is the uncontrolled growth of abnormal cells in the lungs. Lung cancers can start in the cells lining the bronchi, bronchioles, alveoli, or the trachea. As a tumor increases in size, it eventually impairs lung function, causing breathing difficulty, coughing, or pain. Because of the lungs' relatively large size, though, lung cancer can grow undetected for many years. In fact, lung cancer can spread outside the lungs without causing any symptoms. Adding to the confusion, people often mistake the most common symptom of lung cancer, a persistent cough, for a cold or bronchitis.

By the time most people start to notice symptoms serious enough to send them to the doctor, the lung cancer has often grown to be quite large and has spread to the lymph nodes in the chest and perhaps to other parts of the body. Lung cancer can spread by growth of the main tumor, by travel through lymph channels to lymph nodes, or by travel through the bloodstream to other parts of the body.

• • • *Fast Fact* • • •

According to the U.S. Department of Health and Human Services, 87 percent of lung, trachea, and bronchus cancer cases are associated with tobacco use. In the United States, there are 90 million current and former smokers, many of whom are at high risk for lung cancer.

• • •

The Leading Cause of Cancer Death

Take one glance at lung cancer statistics, and it's impossible to breathe easy. The disease is a major public health problem that will kill more people this year than breast cancer, prostate cancer, colon cancer, liver cancer, kidney cancer, and melanoma *combined.*

In 2009, more than 219,000 people in the United States will be diagnosed with new cases of lung cancer. Each year, lung cancer accounts for about 15 percent of all cancer diagnoses in America. Lung cancer is the second most common cancer among men after prostate cancer. Among women, it's the second most common cancer after breast cancer, but lung cancer will kill three times as many men as prostate cancer and nearly twice as many women as breast cancer. Approximately one-third of male cancer deaths and one-quarter of female cancer deaths are due to lung cancer. In fact, since 1987, more women have died of lung cancer each year than from breast cancer. Nearly 160,000 Americans will die of lung cancer in 2009, accounting for about 28 percent of all cancer deaths.

Lung cancer has one of the poorest prognoses of all cancers. Almost three-fourths of people diagnosed with lung cancer die within two years, and at the five-year mark, only 15 percent are still alive. By comparison, today 88 percent of women treated for breast cancer will still be alive five years later. For men with prostate cancer, the five-year survival rate is 99 percent.

Lung cancer is more common among older men and women. In men, it becomes the leading cause of cancer-related death from age 40 onward. In women, it surpasses breast cancer in the group aged 60 and older. In recent years, the incidence of lung cancer in men has been steadily declining, dropping from a high of 102 cases per 100,000 men in 1984 to 73 cases per 100,000 men in 2005. The incidence rate for women has started to level off after climbing for many years. The differences in these trends reflect both historic differences in cigarette smoking between men and women and the overall decrease in smoking rates since the 1970s.

The United States isn't the only country battling lung cancer. Lung cancer has been the most common cancer in the world since 1985. In 2002, about 1.35 million people were diagnosed with lung cancer, and about 1.18 million died of it, making lung cancer the biggest cancer killer in the world. While lung cancer cases have been dropping in the United States and most of Europe as people quit smoking, in the rest of the world, tobacco use continues at high levels, especially among men. In China, for example, cigarette smoking is more popular than ever. Today there are more smokers in China than there are people in the United States, setting the stage for a huge epidemic of lung cancer and other smoking-related diseases there in years to come.

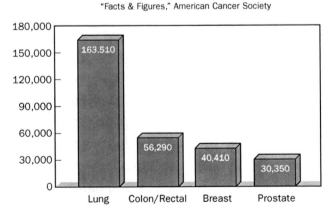

Estimated Mortality of Lung Cancer in 2005
"Facts & Figures," American Cancer Society

Risk Factors for Lung Cancer

By far the single largest risk factor for getting lung cancer is exposure to tobacco smoke. Harmful substances in tobacco smoke damage the cells of the lungs, especially the thin layer of cells that line the bronchi. The cells stop reproducing normally and become cancerous. The greater and longer your exposure to tobacco smoke, the greater your risk. Even people who never smoke are at risk if they're exposed to secondhand smoke from people around them. Although about 87 percent of all lung cancer cases trace back to tobacco use, only about one in ten smokers will develop lung cancer. That doesn't mean the others are safe from tobacco-related disease. Tobacco smoke is the culprit behind many other types of cancer, such as cancer of the esophagus and bladder cancer. It's also the cause of lung diseases such as emphysema and chronic bronchitis, along with heart disease and circulatory problems. Tobacco kills some 400,000 Americans every year.

Some other risk factors for lung cancer aren't directly related to tobacco use, although smokers who are exposed to them have a greater risk than nonsmokers. Nontobacco risk factors include the following:

- **Radon.** Radon is an invisible, odorless, tasteless gas that is a natural decay product of uranium. It forms in soil and rocks—it's everywhere in very low levels. In higher levels, however, radon damages lung cells. People who are exposed to it are at an increased risk of lung cancer, especially if they're smokers. Radon exposure is the second leading cause of lung cancer in the United States and is associated with 15,000 to 22,000 lung cancer deaths each year. The EPA estimates that 1 out of every 15 homes in the United States contains dangerous levels of radon gas (more than 4 picocuries per liter), which can be detected with simple test kits. Radon problems can be easily corrected; once the problem is fixed, the hazard is gone for good.

- **Asbestos and other industrial carcinogens.** A carcinogen is any substance that causes an increased risk of cancer from exposure to it. Asbestos is a well-known carcinogen, which is why it has been removed from buildings and isn't used much industrially any more. For decades, however, asbestos was used in insulation, fire-proofing, and siding for buildings and in many industries. Asbestos fibers tend to break easily into particles that can float in the air and stick to clothes. When the particles are inhaled, they can lodge in the lungs, damaging cells and increasing the risk for lung cancer and mesothelioma, or cancer in the lining of the lungs (the pleura). Carcinogens such as asbestos, arsenic, chromium, nickel, diesel exhaust, soot, tar, and other substances can all cause lung cancer. The risk is highest for those with years of exposure. Overall, the risk from these substances is even higher for smokers.

- **Air pollution.** The risk of lung cancer goes up slightly among people exposed to air pollution; it's responsible for less than 1 percent of all cases. The risk is greater for smokers.

- **Family health history.** Having a father, mother, brother, or sister who had lung cancer puts you at slightly more risk of the disease, even if you don't smoke.

- **Personal health history.** People who have had lung cancer are at increased risk of developing a second lung tumor. Radiation to the chest to treat other cancers, such as lymphoma, puts you at higher risk for lung cancer, especially if you smoke. Chronic obstructive pulmonary disease (COPD), such as emphysema or chronic bronchitis, also increases your risk of lung cancer. The worse your lung function as a result of these diseases, the greater your risk.

- **Gender.** Though the statistics continue to be debated, women appear to have a higher baseline risk of developing lung cancer, as well as a greater susceptibility to the effects of smoking. Differences in how women respond to tobacco-related carcinogens, and possibly the effect of hormone differences, may account for the increased susceptibility.

- **Ethnicity.** Among African American men who smoke, the rate of lung cancer is about 45 percent higher than for white men who smoke.

- **Age.** Two out of three people diagnosed with lung cancer are over age 65; the average age at time of diagnosis is 71. Fewer than 3 percent of all cases are found in people under age 45.

- **Diet and exercise.** Some evidence suggests that a diet low in fruits and vegetables might increase the risk of lung cancer in smokers. According to a recent World Health Organization study, eating the equivalent of at least four cups of vegetables and fruits daily could reduce lung cancer worldwide by 12 percent. Other studies suggest that people who are physically active may have a lower risk of lung cancer than those who aren't, even after taking cigarette smoking into account.

Smoking: The Leading Cause of Lung Cancer

While smoking rates have declined since the U.S. Surgeon General's 1964 *Report on Smoking and Health,* one thing is unchanged: most cases of lung cancer are still connected to smoking. Of course, not all smokers get lung cancer, and some nonsmokers do. But if smoking disappeared tomorrow, lung cancer would cease to be the leading cause of cancer deaths in the United States and the second-most prevalent cause of death—not just from cancer but from any cause—among American men.

It's a frustrating irony that one of the deadliest forms of cancer is also one of the most preventable. People have known about the link between smoking and lung cancer ever since a major study of British doctors who smoked was published in 1956. But today, despite the well-known fact that smoking causes lung cancer, 25 percent of adult men and 20 percent of adult women in the U.S. still smoke.

Smoking accounts for about 87 percent of lung cancer cases in the United States—90 percent in men and

African Americans and Lung Cancer

Lung cancer is the second most common cancer among African American men and women, and it kills more African Americans than any other cancer.

Among African American and Caucasian women, lung cancer rates are about the same. For African American men, however, the rate of lung cancer is about 45 percent higher than among white men. The reasons for this are still unclear, but it's possible that African American men are more susceptible to the carcinogens in cigarette smoke. Lung cancer death rates have been higher among African American men than white men since the 1960s. Overall, African Americans are more likely to die of lung cancer. Paralleling lung cancer rates overall, the rate of lung cancer cases appears to be dropping among African American men in the United States. It continues to rise among African American women.

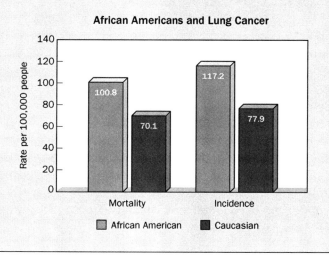

African Americans and Lung Cancer

79 percent in women. Smokers are 8 to 20 times more likely to develop lung cancer compared to people who have never smoked. Plain and simple, smoking cigarettes causes lung

Women and Lung Cancer

Ask most people what cancer is the leading killer of women, and they're likely to say breast cancer. They'd be wrong. In 1987, lung cancer surpassed breast cancer as the leading cause of cancer deaths in women. The overall mortality rate for lung cancer rose steadily throughout the 1980s and peaked around 1990. The incidence of lung cancer peaked in men in 1984 at 86.5 cases per 100,000 men and has been slowly declining ever since. In women, though, the incidence increased during the 1990s and only started to level off starting around 2000. The difference is probably due to the rising ratio of female to male smokers—until the 1950s, most women didn't smoke.

In 2006, Dana Reeve, widow of actor Christopher Reeve, died of lung cancer despite never having smoked. In fact, about 13 percent of lung cancer cases occur among people who have never smoked. We know that exposure to second-hand smoke is a major risk factor among never-smokers and that women who are never-smokers have a higher risk of developing lung cancer than men who are never-smokers. Never-smoking women usually have a type of lung cancer called adenocarcinoma. They tend to be more responsive to treatment, especially with the new targeted therapies, and have a somewhat better long-term outlook. Although some experts think the number of never-smoking women getting lung cancer is going up, the evidence for this isn't clear. The risk of lung cancer in women who have never smoked remains quite low—the risk is about the same as that of getting cervical cancer, which is diagnosed in about 11,000 women each year.

cancer. Surprisingly, nicotine, the main addictive chemical in tobacco, doesn't cause cancer. Cigarette smoke contains a lot more than nicotine, however. Some 4,000 different chemicals are in cigarette smoke. More than 200 of them are poisonous, and more than 40 of them are known to cause cancer.

The longer a person has been smoking and the more packs per day smoked, the greater the risk of lung cancer—and of other smoking-related diseases, such as emphysema. The likelihood that a smoker will develop lung cancer is also affected by the age at which smoking began (younger is worse), and the age at which they quit.

• • • *Fast Fact* • • •

The more cigarettes you've smoked in your lifetime, the greater your risk of lung cancer and other smoking-related diseases. Doctors calculate your risk based in part on your "pack years"—the number of packs of cigarettes you smoked each day times how many years you smoked. So if you smoked 2 packs (40 cigarettes) a day for 20 years, your pack years would be 40. If you smoked half a pack (10 cigarettes) a day for 20 years, your pack years would be 10.

• • •

There's no question that smoking is dangerous to your health and that quitting lowers your risk not only of lung cancer but of many other health problems, such as heart disease, emphysema, and other types of cancer, including bladder cancer. We go into the details and suggest ways that can help you quit in appendix 1—Quit Smoking Now!—at the back of this book.

Moving Forward

Lung cancer can strike current smokers, people who quit years ago, and even people who have never smoked. The cause is less important than getting an accurate diagnosis and beginning treatment. In the next chapter, you'll learn about how lung cancer is diagnosed and staged. In the chapters after that, you'll learn about how lung cancer is treated and the promising new developments that give us hope for even better treatments in the future.

Chapter 2

Diagnosing Lung Cancer

F or most people, lung cancer is discovered in one of two ways: it either causes symptoms that make you go to the doctor to be checked, or it's found when your chest is imaged for some other reason, such as having a chest x-ray taken before you have heart surgery. In this chapter, I'll discuss the symptoms that could mean you have lung cancer and the types of tests that are used to help confirm a diagnosis of lung cancer.

Lung Cancer Symptoms

Most people with lung cancer go to their doctor because they have a new symptom or a change in a symptom that they have had for a long time. Unfortunately, people with lung cancer often don't develop symptoms until their cancer has advanced. At that point, the symptoms can be caused by the tumor pushing on structures within the lung, the spread of the cancer to other areas within the chest, or the spread of the cancer to areas outside of the chest. In addition, the tumor can produce hormonelike substances, which travel through-out the body to cause symptoms outside the lungs, or the body can react to the presence of the tumor in a manner that seems unrelated to the lungs.

The most common symptoms that someone with lung cancer will describe are coughing, shortness of breath, chest pain, fatigue, and/or weight loss. Many other health problems, such as emphysema, heart failure, and heartburn (gastroesophageal reflux disease, or GERD), can cause similar symptoms. To determine if they might be caused by lung cancer, see your doctor if you have any of these symptoms:

- A new cough that doesn't get better over the course of several weeks or an old cough that gets worse

- Shortness of breath beyond what's normal for you and that doesn't improve over the course of several weeks

- A new chest pain that is constant and getting worse over time or is a worsening of a chronic pain

- Fatigue that is constant and getting worse and pre-venting you from carrying out your normal activities

- Unintentional weight loss—that is, your weight is going down even though you're not on a diet

Other, more severe symptoms may develop as the can-cer advances. You may cough up blood, develop debilitating shortness of breath, have very severe chest pain, or have pain in areas of your body that don't seem to be related to your lungs. You may start having headaches or even a seizure.

These symptoms may occur because of a buildup of fluid in the chest between the outer lining of the lungs and the chest wall (pleural effusion), the cancer may have blocked an airway, which can lead to the collapse of part or all of a lung, or the cancer may have spread to other parts of the body and be causing symptoms there.

Paraneoplastic Syndromes

Sometimes, people with lung cancer have a constellation of symptoms and signs that aren't the usual ones for lung cancer. They may seem to be entirely unrelated to the lungs. Known as paraneoplastic syndromes, they can lead to symptoms even before the primary tumor is big enough to be detected. Paraneoplastic syndromes develop either because the tumor produces a substance that activates another part of the body (paraneoplastic endocrine syndromes) or the body develops a reaction to the tumor that interferes with the normal functioning of a distant part of the body (paraneoplastic neurologic syndromes).

Paraneoplastic endocrine syndromes occur when the tumor produces a hormone in an uncontrolled manner; the hormone is similar to one that would normally be produced in a controlled manner by a normal gland in the body. This can result in abnormal levels of sodium and calcium in the body or abnormal production of the body's natural steroid hormones. Symptoms related to these changes include nausea, an altered level of alertness, or even seizures. Problems with the rhythm of the heart can be dangerous.

Paraneoplastic neurologic syndromes occur when the body's response to the tumor affects the functioning of part of the nervous system (brain and nerves). Symptoms can include weakness, changes in sensation, and seizures. Other paraneoplastic syndromes can affect the bones, blood, kidneys, and general well-being. Treating the underlying tumor usually helps relieve the symptoms.

Lung Nodules and Masses

A picture of your lungs—a chest x-ray or CT scan—may be taken to try to explain your symptoms. The image will show abnormal spots in the lungs. If the spot is small (three centimeters or less), it's called a lung nodule. If it's larger than three centimeters, it's called a lung mass.

Chest x-rays will commonly detect a lung nodule as small as one centimeter (a little under half an inch), while chest CT scans can find nodules as small as a couple of millimeters in size, too small to be seen on a chest x-ray. Pictures of the chest may also show other features of lung cancer, including swollen lymph nodes or fluid surrounding the lung.

Lung nodules can be present for many different reasons that aren't lung cancer. A lung nodule may occur after the body has healed from a lung infection or an exposure to something you have breathed in. A lung nodule may also be related to an inflammatory disease, such as rheumatoid arthritis. A lung mass is much more likely to be lung cancer, but it too can be related to any of the same causes of lung nodules.

Your doctor will consider several things when determining how likely it is that your lung nodule or mass represents a lung cancer. Your age, history of smoking, current symptoms, and history of previous cancers all influence the likelihood of cancer. Your doctor will ask about exposures to other risks factors for lung cancer, such as secondhand smoke and asbestos. The doctor will also consider your family history of cancer.

Features of the nodule seen on chest imaging also help your doctor make the diagnosis. It would be very reassuring to see that the nodule was present on a prior picture of the lungs and has not grown since then. A lack of growth for two years or more strongly suggests that the nodule is not cancer. Similarly, if the nodule has gathered calcium in it (this shows up as white on the x-ray or CT scan), it is unlikely to be a cancer.

The larger a nodule is and the more irregular its edges are, the greater the likelihood that cancer is present, especially if the nodule is located in the upper parts of your lung. When a nodule is large enough to be suspicious, its features, along with some additional tests, will be used to determine if cancer is present.

When a nodule is quite small, such as those seen on a chest CT but not a chest x-ray, the chance that it's cancer is quite low. The features discussed above and the tests listed below may not be very accurate for these small nodules. Your doctor may suggest that the best course is just to follow the nodule with scans taken over time. If the nodule grows, your doctor will suggest further action be taken to determine its cause.

Diagnosing Lung Cancer

Diagnosing lung cancer, particularly in the earlier stages, can be challenging. Fortunately, many tests are available to help your doctor determine whether or not lung cancer is present.

Blood Tests

There is currently no blood test available to diagnose lung cancer. Routine blood tests may be performed to help find a different cause of a symptom you're having. Anemia, for instance, can make you feel very tired. Blood tests may also be ordered after lung cancer has been diagnosed to help determine if the cancer has spread to other parts of the body. (This will be discussed more in chapter 3 on staging lung cancer.)

Additional Imaging Tests

If your doctor is concerned about the appearance of your lung nodule, you may be sent for a PET (positron emission tomography) scan. This test is a little more complicated and takes longer than a CT scan, but it's still easy and painless. Before the test, a very small amount of radioactive glucose is injected into your bloodstream. Because cancer cells are more active than normal cells, they absorb more of the radioactive glucose. For the imaging part of the test, you lie on a table that slides slowly through the center of a doughnut-shaped scanner, which detects the radiation and turns it into an image. Brighter spots on the image suggest areas of cancer. PET scans can be very helpful for seeing if the cancer has spread to lymph nodes or other parts of the body. Today, new equipment combines PET and CT scans to give an even better picture of the cancer.

PET scans are very good tests, but they're not perfect. The PET scan pictures will be bright in areas of inflammation or infection, not just cancer. If your PET image shows a bright spot, your doctor will arrange for a biopsy (see below) to investigate further, if it's safe to do so. Sometimes a PET scan can look normal even if cancer is present, especially if the nodule is too small to be detected (under one centimeter) or if the cancer is very slow growing.

Invasive Tests

The only way to know for sure if you have lung cancer is to get a sample of cells or tissue from the lung (or another location of concern identified by imaging) and look at them under a microscope to detect the abnormal cells of cancer. Removing cells or tissues is called a biopsy. The doctor who examines the sample to see if cancer is present is called a pathologist—a doctor who specializes in identifying diseases from biopsies by using a microscope or other techniques to look at the cells. A biopsy is an invasive procedure because your body has to be entered in some way—by a needle, for example—to get the sample.

Samples can be collected in a number of ways, and your doctor may order more than one test to get them. Generally speaking, if you need invasive tests to find possible lung cancer, your primary care doctor will send you to a pulmonologist (a lung specialist) to perform them. In some cases, you may need to see an interventional radiologist (a doctor who specializes in needle biopsy diagnosis guided by imaging) or a thoracic surgeon (a surgeon who specializes in treating the chest area).

Which invasive test you have will depend in part on what your doctor sees on the images of your chest. The list below is alphabetical—which tests are most important and appropriate varies from patient to patient.

Bronchoscopy. For this test, a very thin, flexible tube (a bronchoscope) with a light and a video chip on the end is inserted through the nose or mouth and snaked down into the bronchi. The doctor can then visually examine the airways. Using tiny tools passed through the bronchoscope, the doctor can collect samples from the area of concern. Bronchoscopy is usually done in a pulmonologist's office—you probably won't need to be hospitalized. You're given a short-acting sedative during the procedure to ensure your comfort. Typically, you don't feel anything and wake up quickly afterward. The main risks from this procedure are bleeding and collapse of the lung (pneumothorax) that is biopsied. The risk of complications is low—they occur only in around 1 percent of all bronchoscopies—and they are usually quite easy to manage if they do occur. The chance of getting a diagnosis from bronchoscopy is higher if the area of concern is larger and closer to the center of the lung, where it is easier for the camera to reach. Also, if the scans show a small airway leading to the spot, the doctor will have a better chance of reaching it. An additional benefit of bronchoscopy is that swollen lymph nodes can be sampled at the same time. Modern advances in bronchoscopy tools help to guide the doctor to the worrisome lesions, improving the chance that they can be reached and sampled.

Fine Needle Aspiration or Fine Needle Biopsy (FB). In this technique, the doctor uses a thin needle inserted into a lymph node that can be felt under the skin. Fine needle aspiration can only be used if the tumor or lymph node is easy to feel. Local anesthesia is used, making the procedure painless.

Mediastinoscopy. To get a good look at the mediastinum (the area in your chest between your lungs), the surgeon makes an incision at the top of your breastbone (sternum) and inserts a thin, flexible tube called a mediastinoscope. The tube has a light and a lens on the end, so mediastinoscopy lets the surgeon see the area behind your breastbone and around your heart; tools inserted through the end of the scope let the surgeon take biopsy samples of lymph nodes in the center of the chest. Mediastinoscopy is done under anesthesia in an operating room in a hospital. You can usually go home the same day.

Sputum Cytology. Sputum is a thick fluid that you cough up from the lungs. The sputum can contain cancer cells that can be seen under the microscope. To help you cough up the sputum, the doctor may have you breathe in a mist of salty water. This test is easy and painless; it's done in the doctor's office. It is important that the sputum come from deep in your lungs and is not just spit from the mouth. It is uncommon to diagnose lung cancer from sputum cytology.

Thoracentesis. If you have a lot of fluid around your lungs, the doctor uses a long, thin needle inserted through the skin of your back to remove it. The lab checks the fluid for cancer cells. This test is done in the doctor's office with local anesthesia so you don't feel anything as the needle is inserted.

Thoracoscopy. In this surgical procedure, the surgeon makes several small incisions into your chest and uses a thin, flexible thoracoscope with a light and a lens on the end to look at the lungs and nearby tissues. A tool on the end of the thoracoscope can be used to biopsy suspicious-looking tissues. Thoracoscopy is often done under general anesthesia in an operating room at a hospital.

Thoracotomy. The surgeon opens your chest with a long incision to get a good view. Lymph nodes and other tissue samples are usually removed. Thoracotomy is done under general anesthesia in an operating room in a hospital. You usually have to stay in the hospital for a day or two or possibly longer afterward.

Transthoracic Needle Biopsy (TNB). This procedure is used to get a sample from a tumor or lymph node that's deeper in the chest and harder to reach. Under the guidance of a CT scan, x-ray, or ultrasound, the doctor inserts a needle through the chest wall and lung into the abnormal area to get a sample of tissue. There is a slightly higher risk of a collapsed lung (pneumothorax) from this procedure than there is for bronchoscopy. You may be given a short-acting sedative so you won't feel anything and will wake up quickly afterward. You can usually go home the same day. This procedure has a better chance of getting an answer if the abnormal area is very close to the edge of the lung.

Which Procedure Is Best for Me?

Your doctor will consider several factors when deciding which procedure is the best one for you. The location and size of the tumor are important in deciding if a bronchoscopy or transthoracic needle biopsy is more likely to be able to reach it. It may be possible to get information about the spread of the cancer with bronchoscopy or mediastinoscopy if the lymph nodes in the center of the chest are swollen. If the cancer appears to be in a very early stage, it may be possible to remove it through a thoracoscopy or thoracotomy. Thoracentesis is only useful if fluid is seen surrounding the lung. Your general health and the expertise of your local

Questions to Ask about Biopsies

A biopsy is crucial for determining if you have lung cancer and, if so, what to do next. You and your doctor will need to work together on what biopsy procedure is best for you. To help you decide, ask your doctor these questions:

- Which procedure do you recommend? How is the tissue removed?
- Will I need to stay in the hospital? If so, for how long?
- What do I need to do to prepare for the procedure?
- How long will it take? Will I be awake? Will it hurt?
- What are the risks of complications, such as a collapsed lung?
- How long will it take me to recover?
- When will I know the results?

doctors with these tests will influence the risks and benefits of each procedure. Feel free to have a conversation with your doctor about the reason a certain test is being chosen over another one.

Screening for Lung Cancer

Screening means trying to find a disease before the disease has caused any symptoms to suggest it is there. The goal of screening is to detect the disease early enough in its course that it can be cured. Ultimately, a screening program is only successful if it reduces the number of deaths due to that disease (in this case lung cancer) in the group that receives the screening test.

Many studies have tried to find a good screening test for lung cancer. These have included tests looking for cancer in the sputum, on chest x-rays, and on CT scans. The individuals included in these studies were those who were felt to be at a high risk of developing lung cancer (for example, people who have a significant history of smoking). Unfortunately, none of the screening studies performed so far have been able to show fewer lung cancer deaths in the group that received the screening test compared to the group that didn't. Currently, none of the major lung organizations or cancer societies recommendss lung cancer screening. Despite this, the topic of lung cancer screening is one of the most debated areas in academic medicine. While some feel we should be screening people now, most feel that we should wait for the results of several ongoing large studies that are looking at CT screening for lung cancer. These results should be available within the next few years. In addition, new methods of screening, including blood and breath testing for lung cancer, are being developed. Whether these will ultimately prove to be useful tests remain to be seen. If you're concerned about your risk of lung cancer, discuss the pros and cons of screening it for with your lung specialist.

• • • *Fast Fact* • • •

For the approximately 15 percent of people with lung cancer who don't go to the doctor with symptoms, their lung cancer generally is discovered on a chest x-ray or CT scan performed for some other reason.

• • •

The Symptoms of Lung Cancer

About 85 percent of patients with lung cancer have some symptoms when they go to their doctors.

SYMPTOM	PERCENTAGE OF PEOPLE WHO HAVE SYMPTOM
Cough	46
Weight loss	32
Shortness of breath	30
Chest pain	30
Fever	28
Coughing up blood	27
No symptom	15

The Next Steps

The samples from a biopsy are examined under a microscope by a pathologist. The pathology report will be sent to all the doctors who are treating you, but you will probably discuss the results with your pulmonologist.

The pathology report will say what type of lung cancer you have. The two most common forms are non–small cell lung cancer (NSCLC) and small cell lung cancer (SCLC). There are different types of cancer within those categories, and the pathology report will indicate which type you have.

The pathology report, along with the results from your other scans and tests, helps your doctor decide the stage of your cancer, or how far along and serious it is. Accurate staging is extremely important for deciding on your treatment plan going forward. In fact, it's so important that we'll spend the next chapter discussing the different kinds of lung cancer and how they're staged.

Chapter 3

Types and Staging of Lung Cancer

ung cancer is divided into two main types: non–small
cell lung cancer (NSCLC) and small cell lung cancer
(SCLC). The two types of lung cancer are quite distinct in their presentation, prognosis, and treatment. Once
lung cancer is suspected, deciding what type you have and
how far it has progressed—what stage it has reached—is
crucial for deciding what treatment will be best for you. In
this chapter, we'll look at both types of cancer, explain how
they're staged, and help you understand what staging means
for your treatment decisions going forward.

Non–Small Cell Lung Cancer

Non–small cell lung cancer gets its name because under the microscope, the cancerous cells appear large and irregular. NSCLC accounts for nearly 85 percent of all lung cancer cases. Within NSCLC, the cancer cells can take many different forms, but most fall into three basic categories. Which type of NSCLC you have depends on how the cells look under the microscope. To decide, a pathologist will examine cells taken from you during a biopsy.

Adenocarcinoma

Adenocarcinoma means a cancer that's found in a tissue that secretes something—in the case of your lungs, it's found in the mucus-secreting epithelial cells that line the bronchi. This form of lung cancer is often found in the lung's outer edges, in the smaller airways. Adenocarcinoma accounts for about 40 percent of lung cancer cases in the United States. It's the most common type of lung cancer overall for both men and women, and it's the most common type in people who never smoked.

Adenocarcinoma often spreads to the spaces between the lungs and the chest wall. Its location means that most people don't have any symptoms in the early stages. It's not uncommon for an adenocarcinoma to be discovered incidentally when someone has a chest x-ray or CT scan for some other reason. Adenocarcinoma of the lung has a highly variable presentation and course. In some people, it grows rapidly and aggressively, spreading quickly to other parts of the body,

while in other people, the cancer can be very slow growing. Particularly in women who have never smoked, adenocarcinoma may grow more slowly and be fairly responsive
to treatment, especially with targeted therapies, leading to
longer survival.

Squamous Cell Carcinoma

Squamous cell carcinoma originates in the thin, flat cells that
line the passages of the respiratory tract. *Squamous* in medical
terminology means scalelike, and these cells do look a bit like
fish scales. This type of NSCLC accounts for about 30 percent
of lung cancer cases in the United States. While the tumor is
still small, this type of lung cancer can be difficult to detect
on x-rays and CT scans, because the cancer may be inside the
airways, not out in the lung tissue.

In recent years, the number of patients in the United
States with squamous cell lung cancers has steadily decreased.
This may be because of the advent of filtered and "light" cigarettes, which have led to people actually inhaling the smoke
more deeply into their lungs, where it can cause adenocarcinoma instead.

Large Cell Carcinomas

Large cell carcinomas make up a group of cancers that look
large and rounded under a microscope and may begin in
several types of large cells. This cancer is usually found in the
outer edges of the lung. Sometimes called undifferentiated
carcinoma, it's the least common type of NSCLC. Mixtures
of different types of NSCLC cells are also sometimes seen.

Mesothelioma

Mesothelioma is a rare form of cancer that affects the mesothelium, a protective membrane that covers most of the body's internal organs. The mesothelium has two layers, one that surrounds an organ and another that forms a sac around it. A lubricating fluid fills the space between the two membranes and makes moving organs, such as your lungs, able to glide easily against other organs, blood vessels, muscles, and so on. Depending on the part of the body the mesothelium covers, it has different names. The part that surrounds the lungs and lines the wall of the chest cavity is called the pleura; the part that covers and protects the heart is called the pericardium.

Cancer can sometimes arise in the mesothelium, usually in the pleura or pericardium but sometimes in the abdominal area. Mesothelioma, as this cancer is called, usually happens decades after exposure to asbestos. About 70 to 80 percent of people with mesothelioma have a history of working with asbestos—in a shipyard, a cement factory, or an industrial site making brakes or textiles, for example. However, most people exposed to asbestos never get mesothelioma, and some people who get mesothelioma have never worked with asbestos. This rare cancer affects only about 2,000 people a year.

Mesothelioma can be hard to diagnose. The symptoms include shortness of breath and chest pain, symptoms that can easily be mistaken for other health problems, such as bronchitis. As with lung cancer, the diagnostic steps include physical exam, imaging, blood tests, and a biopsy. The treatment for mesothelioma confined to the pleura on a healthy person is surgery. The surgery means removal of all of the affected lung. Sometimes part of the diaphragm is also removed. Very often, however, the cancer is too advanced for surgery. Radiation and chemotherapy are also used to treat mesothelioma, whether or not the patient has surgery.

Carcinoid Lung Tumors

Carcinoid lung tumors are rare, slow-growing tumors. Only about 1 to 2 percent of all cancers in the lung are carcinoids—only about 3,000 people are diagnosed with this disease every year in the United States. Carcinoid lung tumors occur somewhat more often in women than in men. They usually occur when the person is around the age of 60, which is slightly younger than average for lung cancer, but these tumors have been found in people of all ages, even children. Surprisingly, smoking and exposure to tobacco smoke aren't related to carcinoid lung tumors. We don't really know what the risk factors are.

About nine out of ten people with this tumor have typical carcinoids. These tumors grow slowly and only rarely spread beyond the lung. Atypical carcinoids grow a bit faster and are somewhat more likely to spread beyond the lungs to other organs.

The treatment is to remove the tumor surgically if it can be reached that way—and fortunately, most carcinoid lung tumors are operable. In most cases, removing the tumor is all that's needed to cure the patient. For patients who can't have surgery, either because the tumor can't be reached or because their overall health is poor, radiation therapy can be used if the tumor has not spread, and chemotherapy plus radiation therapy would be considered if the tumor has spread.

Staging Non–Small Cell Lung Cancer

Once your doctor has determined what type of non–small cell lung cancer you have, the next crucial step is staging—learning if the cancer has spread within the lungs or to other parts

Premalignant Lesions

A premalignant lesion in the lung is an area where the cells show abnormal growth that could become cancerous. Premalignant adenocarcinoma lesions appear as what are called ground-glass opacities on a CT scan. The lesions are very small, usually under five millimeters (about three-eighths of an inch), and haven't invaded the surrounding tissue. They are called atypical adenomatous hyperplasia. Squamous cell premalignant lesions occur in the lining cells of the airways (termed squamous dysplasia). They can generally only be seen with bronchoscopy techniques.

Because the majority of lung cancer patients already have advanced stage lung cancer by the time they are diagnosed, finding ways to spot and treat premalignant lesions, before they have time to turn into true malignancies is a major research goal. Chemoprevention—using drugs, supplements, and other substances—is one approach, but so far there haven't been any real breakthroughs. In fact, one promising substance called beta carotene turned out actually to increase the incidence of lung cancer in people who where already at high risk. The best prevention we have now is to stop smoking and avoid tobacco smoke.

of the body. What stage your cancer has reached will help you and your doctor decide what your treatment will be.

As part of the diagnosis process, your cancer has already been clinically staged based on your physical exam, imaging tests, and blood work. Your doctor probably has a good idea of whether the cancer has spread beyond your lung to the other lung, any nearby lymph nodes, and other organs.

If you've had a biopsy to obtain a sample of the cancer, a pathologist will look carefully at the cells under a microscope to see what type of cancer you have. Biopsy of the primary tumor contributes to the staging, but other factors also have to be considered, including the imaging findings and biopsies of other suspicious sites, such as lymph nodes. Surgical staging happens when a patient has a lung resection for treatment. At that point the surgeon can remove additional tissue and more lymph nodes for examination by the pathologist. Surgical staging may show that the cancer is more extensive than could be detected from imaging and other tests.

Staging NSCLC is a bit complicated, but it's important to understand the way it works so that you can communicate effectively with all your doctors. Staging NSCLC is based on the TNM classification system developed by the American Joint Committee on Cancer (AJCC) in 1986 and updated in 1997 and again in 2009. This system replaces older staging systems and is now used by all doctors, which means that no matter where you are diagnosed, the staging system will be the same.

In the TNM system, each non–small cell lung cancer is assigned a *T, N,* and *M* category:

- *T* stands for the primary tumor.
- *N* stands for spread to lymph nodes.
- *M* stands for metastasis (spread to other parts of the body).

Let's take a closer look at each category.

T: Analyzing the Primary Tumor

Each patient's T value describes the size and level of invasion into the lung's nearby structures. The higher the T number, the larger the size of the tumor, and the more it may have grown into nearby structures:

- **Tis:** Cancer is found only in the layer of cells lining the air passages. It has not invaded other lung tissues. This stage is also known as carcinoma in situ.

- **T0:** No primary tumor is present.

- **T1:** The cancer is no larger than three centimeters along its longest portion (slightly less than one and one-fourth of an inch, or about the size of a walnut). It hasn't spread to the membranes that surround the lungs (the pleura) and does not affect the main branches of the bronchi.

- **T2:** The cancer has one or more of the following characteristics:
  - It is larger than three centimeters and smaller than seven centimeters.
  - It involves a main bronchus but isn't closer than two centimeters (about three-fourths of an inch) to the main carina, the point where the trachea (windpipe) branches into the left and right main bronchi.
  - It has grown into the membranes that surround the lungs.

- The cancer may partially clog the airways, but this hasn't caused the entire lung to collapse.

- **T3:** The cancer has one or more of the following features:

  - It is larger than seven cm.

  - It has spread to the chest wall, the diaphragm, the membranes surrounding the space between the two lungs (mediastinal pleura), or the membranes of the sac surrounding the heart (parietal pericardium).

  - It has invaded a main bronchus and is closer than two centimeters to the main carina (the point where trachea branches into the left and right main bronchi), but it doesn't affect this area.

  - It has grown into the airways enough to cause an entire lung to collapse.

  - Two or more separate tumor nodules are present in the same lobe of the lung.

- **T4:** The cancer has one or more of the following features:

  - It has spread to the space behind the breastbone (sternum) and in front of the heart (mediastinum), the heart, the windpipe, the esophagus, the backbone, or the point where the windpipe branches into the left and right main bronchi.

  - Two separate areas of the same cancer are present in different lobes within the same lung.

N: Analyzing the Lymph Nodes

Each patient's N value depends on which, if any, of the lymph nodes in or near the lungs are affected by the cancer. The higher the N number, the more involved the lymph nodes are:

- **N0:** No spread to lymph nodes.

- **N1:** Cancer has spread to lymph nodes within the lung or located around the area where the bronchus enters the lung (hilar lymph nodes). The cancer affects lymph nodes only on the same side as the main tumor.

- **N2:** Cancer has spread to lymph nodes in the center of the chest (the mediastinum). The affected lymph nodes are on the same side as the main tumor.

- **N3:** Cancer has spread to lymph nodes near the collarbone on either side or to hilar or mediastinal lymph nodes on the opposite side as the main tumor.

Tumors that are rated N2 or N3 are said to be locally advanced, meaning that the cancer has spread to lymph nodes in the chest region but not beyond.

M: Analyzing Spread to Other Parts of the Body

Each patient's M (metastasis) value depends on whether the cancer has spread to distant tissues and organs:

- **M0:** No spread to distant organs or areas. Sites considered distant include the other lung; lymph nodes farther away than those mentioned in N stages; and other organs or tissues, such as the liver, bones, or brain.

- **M1:** The cancer has spread to one or more distant sites—either to another organ or to the other lung— or a cancerous pleural effusion is present (fluid around the lung). Spread to the other lung or within the fluid around the lung is called M1a, whereas spread to a distant site (brain, bones, liver, and adrenal glands) is considered M1b.

If the cancer has metastasized to distant organs, the patient is said to have advanced or metastatic lung cancer.

Stage Grouping for Non–Small Cell Lung Cancer

Once a patient's T, N, and M values are determined, the information is combined, and an overall stage of lung cancer is assigned. The stages are described using the Roman numerals from I to IV. Stage I cancers are the least advanced, and higher numbers indicate more spread. Generally speaking, the more advanced the cancer is, the worse the outlook.

Stage I and stage II disease are localized—the primary tumor and any involved lymph nodes are contained within one portion of the lung and can be completely removed by surgery.

Stage III disease is locally advanced. The primary tumor has invaded structures that can't be surgically removed, or lymph nodes outside the lobe containing the primary tumor are involved. Locally advanced disease can't be completely resected—in the rare cases were surgery is done, some cancer will still be left behind.

Stage IV disease is metastatic lung cancer. The primary tumor has spread to other parts of the body, most commonly the other lung, brain, bones, liver, or adrenal glands, although it can go anywhere.

Within the main four stages are substages that describe the size and spread of the cancer more precisely. Your doctor will discuss your staging with you in more detail once he or she has all the available information from tests, biopsies, and surgery.

Recurrent non–small cell lung cancer is cancer that has come back after it was first treated. Recurrences may be anywhere in the body. Even when recurrent lung cancer comes back in another organ, it's still called lung cancer.

Staging Tests—Non–Small Cell Lung Cancer

Your doctor will order tests that help determine the stage of your cancer. The tests ordered will be based on your symptoms and the information gathered from tests that have helped to diagnose the cancer. In general, a PET scan is performed to help evaluate for spread within the chest (e.g. lymph nodes in the mediastinum) and outside the chest (e.g. bones, liver, adrenal glands). The only place not seen well by PET imaging is the brain. Thus, if you have symptoms of brain involvement or your cancer appears to be at least locally advanced, a separate brain scan will be ordered (CT or MRI). Lab work may be ordered based on your symptoms as well. Since defining the extent of your disease is so important, findings on the

PET scan or blood work are usually confirmed by additional biopsies whenever possible.

Small Cell Lung Cancer

Small cell lung cancer (SCLC) is much less common than non–small cell lung cancer—only about 15 percent of all lung cancers are the small cell type. This type of cancer is always caused by smoking. It's called small cell lung cancer because under the microscope, the cancer cells are small and are mostly filled up by the cell nucleus (the control center of the cell). Although the cells are small, they can also be very aggressive, reproducing rapidly to form large tumors that spread quickly to the lymph nodes and other parts of the body.

Small cell carcinomas tend to present with a relatively small lung nodule or mass and relatively large hilar and mediastinal lymph nodes. Symptoms of general illness, such as weight loss, are more common. People with SCLC may also have the signs and symptoms of a paraneoplastic syndrome. This means that tumor is producing one or more substances that enter into the bloodstream and cause symptoms that affect other organs. (See chapter 2 for more on this.)

Staging Small Cell Lung Cancer

The tests you have already had, including imaging and biopsy results, have told your doctor that you have small cell lung cancer. The next step is to stage the cancer and determine how far it has spread in your lung and if it has spread to other parts of your body. The staging is very important for helping you and your doctor decide what treatment will be best for you.

Small cell lung cancer has only two stages:

1. Limited-stage disease (LD): The cancer is found only in one lung, in the tissues between the lungs, and only in nearby lymph nodes. About 30 percent of people with SCLC have limited-stage disease at the time of diagnosis.

2. Extensive-stage disease (ED): The cancer has spread outside the lung where it started, or it has spread to other parts of the body, such as the liver, adrenal glands, or brain. About 70 percent of people with SCLC have extensive-stage disease at the time of diagnosis.

The two-stage system used today for staging SCLC replaces older systems that were more complicated but not really more helpful in deciding what treatment should be.

Recurrent small cell lung cancer is cancer that has come back after being treated. The cancer may come back in the chest, brain, or other parts of the body, but it is still small cell lung cancer.

Staging Tests—Small Cell Lung Cancer

Your doctor will order tests to determine the stage of your small cell lung cancer based on your symptoms and the testing that has been performed to help diagnose the cancer. PET imaging may be performed to assess sites of tumor involvement

Questions to Ask about Staging

- What type of lung cancer do I have?
- What stage is the cancer?
- What's the usual prognosis for people with my type and stage of cancer?
- May I have a copy of the pathology report?

within and outside of the chest, though many physicians still use CT scans of the chest, abdomen, and pelvis in addition to bone scans for staging. Brain imaging is mandatory, as there is a higher chance the tumor has spread to the brain. Labwork is often performed to assess for associated conditions.

The Next Step: Treatment

The next step after accurately staging your cancer is to consider your treatment options with your doctor. The type and stage of your cancer are the major factors to think about, but other issues, such as your overall health, enter into the decision. Making the right choices can be complicated, as you'll learn in the next chapter.

Chapter 4

Treating Non–Small Cell Lung Cancer

The next step after diagnosing and staging non–small cell lung cancer is working with your health care team to decide on the best treatment plan for you. The decision can be complex because many factors have to be considered: the stage of your cancer, your overall health, and your personal preferences. Although lung cancer is serious and you don't want any needless delays in beginning treatment, take the time to be sure you understand exactly what the treatment options are and how they will affect you.

Treatment Options for Non–Small Cell Lung Cancer

Three types of standard treatment are used for non–small cell lung cancer. Standard treatments are those that are currently in use for most patients—they're the basic guidelines doctors follow. Because standard treatments become standard only after they've been in use for a while and have been shown to help, doctors know these treatments work well, and they know what to expect from them. Standard treatments are sometimes used alone, but they're more often used in combination—you might have both surgery and radiation therapy, for example.

One size doesn't fit all in lung cancer treatment. Your treatment will be individualized for you and might well differ from what someone else with lung cancer or a different type of cancer receives.

Surgery

The standard surgery for localized lung cancer is a lobectomy, which removes the entire lobe where the main tumor lives. By removing the entire lobe, there's a lower risk of recurrence. If your overall lung function is too poor to tolerate having an entire lobe removed, a limited resection, also known as a wedge or segmental resection, may be done instead. In a limited resection, the cancerous part of the lung lobe is removed along with a small amount of the surrounding healthy tissue. If the tumor or affected lymph nodes are in the central part of the lung, you may need a pneumonectomy, meaning the entire lung is removed. A procedure called a sleeve resection is sometimes done to remove an upper lobe tumor and part of the bronchus in an effort to avoid having to remove the whole lung. Surgeons always try to use the technique that gives you the best chance of curing the cancer, while removing the smallest amount of lung and preserving the most lung capacity.

Most lung cancer surgeries are performed through a thoracotomy, where a large incision is made in the chest wall to let the surgeon see the entire lung. More often nowadays, your surgeon may perform the surgery with smaller incisions and the use of a camera, called a VATS procedure (video-assisted thoracoscopic surgery). This is particularly true if a smaller tumor is being removed. VATS surgery can shorten your recovery time and minimize your discomfort. If not already performed, a mediastinoscopy (surgery to evaluate the lymph nodes in the mediastinum) will often be performed at the start of the lung cancer surgery in an effort to be sure you aren't dealing with more advanced cancer than testing has been able to uncover.

Is Surgery Right for You? Your doctors will help decide if surgery is right for you based on the type and stage of your cancer, as well as your ability to tolerate the surgery and live well afterwards. Surgery for lung cancer is a major operation. The surgery itself has risks, such as internal bleeding and infection, and a very small but real risk of death. If you have surgery, you'll usually be up on your feet in just a couple of days, and you'll probably be home from the hospital in just four to six days. After that, you can resume your normal activities as you feel able—just don't do any heavy lifting for six weeks.

To decide if you're strong enough to tolerate surgery and maintain a good quality of life afterwards, your doctors will need to know how well your lungs work. If part or all of a lung has to be removed, your doctors need to be sure that you will have enough lung capacity left to be able to breathe well. To find out, you may be asked to have some lung function tests, also called pulmonary function tests (PFT).

The main lung function test is called spirometry. This measures how much air you can move in and out of your lungs and how quickly you can do it. The test is usually done in a pulmonologist's office by a respiratory therapist or technician. It's painless and quick. For the test, you'll wear a noseclip and breathe into a mouthpiece attached to a recording device called a spirometer. The information is printed out on a chart called a spirogram.

Other lung function tests may also be needed. Gas diffusion tests, for instance, measure how efficiently oxygen crosses the alveoli (the tiny sacs in your lung) and enters your bloodstream. Other tests measure your capacity for exercise and help to estimate how much of your lung function will be lost with surgery. You may also need to pass a stress test of your heart. Knowledge of the type and stage of your lung cancer and the results of these tests will give your doctors a very good idea of whether surgery is right for you.

Radiation Therapy

In radiation therapy, high-energy protons or other types of radiation are used to kill cancer cells or keep them from growing. External radiation therapy uses a high-tech machine to send a very targeted beam of radiation into your body, aimed at the cancer to avoid damaging surrounding tissue.

If you need standard external beam radiation therapy to the lungs, you will usually have it every day, five days a week, for about six weeks. The treatment itself is painless and quick. Another type of radiation, called stereotactic radiotherapy, is given once a day for only three to five days. (We'll discuss stereotactic radiotherapy more in chapter 7.)

The most common side effect of radiation to the chest is difficulty swallowing due to inflammation of the esophagus (esophagitis). This is usually temporary and goes away quickly once treatment stops. Another common side effect is inflammation of the lung tissue (pneumonitis), which can cause coughing and shortness of breath. The symptoms can be treated with medications. Radiation pneumonitis can sometimes be very serious and permanent.

Chemotherapy

Chemotherapy works by interfering with the ability of cells in your body to divide or reproduce themselves. Cells that grow rapidly—like cancer cells—are strongly affected by chemotherapy drugs. Most of the cells in your body don't grow rapidly, so they're not affected by the drugs. Some cells in your body do reproduce quickly, however, including your bone marrow (where blood cells are made), your hair, and the lining of your intestines. Unfortunately, chemotherapy drugs do affect these cells. The level of your red blood cells, white blood cells, and platelets (tiny particles in your blood important for clotting) may drop because the bone marrow is affected. You may have nausea, vomiting, and diarrhea from the drugs' effects on your gastrointestinal tract. (However, most chemotherapy drugs don't make you lose your hair.) Chemotherapy isn't easy to get through, but today we have a lot of excellent drugs that can help manage the side effects and get you through the treatment with the least possible discomfort (see chapter 6).

When chemotherapy is given after and in addition to surgery for cancer, it's called adjuvant therapy, meaning treatment that's designed to help in the prevention, relief, or cure of disease. Adjuvant chemotherapy for non–small cell lung cancer has been shown to improve five-year survival rates. Adjuvant chemotherapy is most helpful for people with stage II and stage III disease (see below).

Even after years of research, there's no clear agreement among doctors on which chemotherapy drugs are best for lung cancer. The most commonly used chemotherapy is what doctors call a doublet: a platinum-based drug, usually one called cisplatin or carboplatin, along with another drug. There's no clear agreement on what drug is best as the second part of the doublet—studies show that they're all equal. Your oncologist will decide what doublet combination is best for you. Whatever drugs you get, the "cocktail" will also include a drug to help prevent nausea and vomiting; you may also get other drugs to help prevent other side effects. The drugs are given intravenously, usually in around four cycles, each given approximately three weeks apart. Depending on the drug combination, each treatment lasts about three to five hours.

A new class of chemotherapy drugs, called targeted therapy, is now coming into wider use for lung cancer. Medications in this class target abnormal processes in cancer cells. They work more specifically against just the cancer cells. Nothing is perfect, and these treatments are not without side effects. They're such a hopeful development in treating lung

Clinical Trials

Standard treatment is almost always the preferred approach for any type and stage of lung cancer. Many patients, however, also participate in clinical trials, which help advance the science of cancer treatment while also providing top-level care. The purpose of clinical trials is to learn if a new cancer treatment—a new drug, for example—is safe and effective and if it might be better than standard treatment. When you participate in a clinical trial, you usually receive standard treatment plus an additional drug or a different type of radiation therapy. Many of today's standard treatments were developed on the basis of clinical trials. Participating in one may mean that you are among the first to receive a new treatment that could turn out to be helpful.

cancer that we'll talk about them in detail in chapter 7 on advances in treatment.

Treatment Options by Stage

In most cases, your treatment choices will depend on the stage of your cancer, along with your overall state of health. Not every treatment or combination of treatments for a particular stage will necessarily be right for you.

Stage I NSCLC

Whenever possible, standard treatment for patients with stage I NSCLC is surgery, usually a lobectomy. For most patients at this stage, no further treatment is needed, and the five-year survival rate is between 60 and 80 percent. For patients who can't have surgery because of other health problems or who choose not to have surgery, the standard treatment is external beam radiation. While this isn't as effective as surgery to remove the cancer, it's more effective than no treatment at all.

Chemotherapy after the surgery isn't usually recommended. If the tumor is quite large, however, it may be considered. Radiation therapy after surgery isn't usually recommended unless the surgeon wasn't able to remove the entire tumor. Whether the treatment is surgery, with or without chemotherapy, or radiation therapy alone, the goal is to cure the cancer.

Stage II NSCLC

For patients with stage II NSCLC cancer, standard treatment is surgery—usually a lobectomy or pneumonectomy—followed by chemotherapy using a platinum-based drug if the patient is well enough to tolerate it. With this treatment, the five-year survival rate is between 40 to 50 percent. For patients who can't have surgery or choose not to, the standard treatment is external beam radiation therapy. The goal of treatment is to cure the cancer, but radiation therapy alone isn't as effective as surgery.

Stage III NSCLC

Stage III NSCLC is a diverse set of conditions. Most stage III cancer is related to involvement of the mediastinal lymph nodes. Some is stage III due to local growth of the tumor alone.

Patients with stage III NSCLC due to lymph node involvement cancer can't have all of their cancer removed by surgery, which makes treatment decisions more complex. The goal of treatment in someone healthy enough to tolerate it is still to cure the cancer, though the odds are not as good as they are for stage I and II.

Standard treatment for stage III lung cancer due to lymph node involvement, in people who are well enough to tolerate it, is concurrent chemoradiotherapy. This means the patient gets chemotherapy using a platinum-based drug and another drug and gets radiation therapy at the same time.

Some very healthy patients with stage IIIa lung cancer may be offered surgery after chemoradiotherapy, ideally as part of a clinical trial. This isn't standard treatment, and it's only done after chemotherapy and radiation therapy have shrunk the tumor. Chemotherapy is usually given afterward as well. Sometimes you are only diagnosed with stage III lung cancer after surgery for what appeared to be a lower-stage cancer. During the surgery, lymph nodes are removed that can show a little bit of cancer in them. In this situation, chemotherapy would be offered after recovering from the surgery.

If a person has stage III cancer because the primary tumor is a T4 (usually meaning it has grown within the chest to invade vital structures), surgery is typically not possible. In this situation, the risks and benefits of radiation and/or chemotherapy will be discussed with you. (See chapter 3 for more on what T4 means.)

Stage IV NSCLC

Stage IV lung cancer means the cancer has spread outside the chest to other areas in the body. At this stage, the goal of treatment is to extend a person's life and maintain the quality of life. For patients well enough to tolerate it, the standard treatment at this stage is chemotherapy with a combination of a platinum-based drug and another drug. Chemotherapy at this stage has been proven to relieve symptoms, improve the quality of life, and prolong survival. Patients who have non–squamous cell cancer may benefit from adding a targeted therapy drug called bevacizumab (Avastin) to standard chemotherapy (see chapter 7 for more on this and similar drugs).

Radiation therapy may also be suggested to treat a metastasis to a bone that's causing pain or is likely to cause the bone to break. Similarly radiation may be helpful if the tumor is invading a large airway leading to symptoms. Other treatments to help open a blocked large airway may also be used, including laser therapy, brachytherapy (inserting a catheter with a radioactive substance in it into the area), electrocautery to burn away the obstruction, and placing a stent (tube) into the airway to prop it open.

Lung cancer can spread to the brain. Radiation therapy is the best treatment for the brain metastasis when this occurs. If there are only one to three brain tumors, a type of radiation machine called a gamma knife may be used to target the tumors and destroy them with a single treatment of very high-dose radiation. (We'll talk more about radiosurgery in chapter 7.) When there are more than three brain metastases, whole-brain radiation therapy is used instead.

Many older patients with advanced lung cancer don't opt for chemotherapy, even though it can help prolong their lives and can be given safely. They think they're too old to cope with chemotherapy, but research has shown that many older patients can manage well—age alone isn't necessarily a reason to avoid this treatment. Your oncologist will choose your treatment drugs based on your overall well-being and other health issues. The goal is to give you the best chance of benefiting from the treatment while minimizing the potential for harm.

Recurrent Non–Small Cell Lung Cancer

If the lung cancer recurs, it often comes back in the other lung or in distant organs, such as the brain. Any of the available treatments (surgery, chemotherapy, and radiation therapy) may be offered at this point. The treatment that's recommended will depend on several factors. The initial stage and type of tumor, the treatments that have already been given, the location of the recurrence, and the person's general health are all considered by the doctor when helping to decide on the best treatment options for recurrent lung cancer.

Performance Status

Many patients with lung cancer also have other lung problems, such as emphysema, heart problems, or both, which make surgery or chemotherapy more difficult or may mean they can't have surgery or chemotherapy at all. To help decide if you'll be able to go through chemotherapy successfully, doctors look at your performance status (PS). They use a rating system called a performance scale. The scale looks at how well you can work, move around, and do all the usual activities of daily living.

Rating Your Performance Status

A widely used performance status rating system is called the Eastern Cooperative Oncology Group (ECOG) Performance Scale. Here's how the rating system works.

Eastern Cooperative Oncology Group (ECOG)
Performance Scale

PERFORMANCE STATUS	DEFINITION
0	Fully active; no performance restriction
1	Strenuous physical activity restricted; fully ambulatory and able to carry out light work
2	Capable of self-care but unable to carry out any work activities; up and about for more than 50 percent of waking hours
3	Capable of only limited self-care; confined to bed or chair more than 50 percent of waking hours
4	Completely disabled; cannot carry out any self-care; totally confined to bed or chair

The higher your rating on the performance scale, the less likely it is you are a good candidate for chemotherapy or surgery.

The Prognosis for Treatment

The long-term outlook—the prognosis—for people with non–small cell lung cancer depends mostly on the stage of the cancer. The best outlook is for people with stage I and stage II tumors that can be removed by surgery. These patients

Your Treatment Team

As you go through treatment for non–small cell lung cancer, you'll be working with a lot of different people. Your treatment team will include the following:

- Your primary care doctor
- Your pulmonologist (lung specialist)
- Your thoracic (chest) surgeon
- Your radiation oncologist (the cancer specialist who directs your radiation therapy)
- Your medical oncologist (the cancer specialist who directs your chemotherapy)

Physician assistants, nurses, respiratory therapists, and radiation technologists will also help with your treatment. You may also need the help of a social worker to arrange for other aspects of your care, such as a home health care aide. It's sometimes hard to know which team member is responsible for what part of your treatment and whom to call if you have a question or problem. Many patients find it helpful to keep a list with all the names and phone numbers of the treatment team. It's also helpful to write down questions before appointments or as they occur to you so you can be sure to get them answered.

can often be cured and remain cancer-free. Among patients at this stage who can't have surgery, radiation therapy may also cure the cancer. For patients with stage II and some stage III disease, chemotherapy after surgery is often helpful for preventing recurrence.

For patients with stage III cancer—where the tumor has spread to the lymph nodes in the middle of the chest or has invaded vital structures within the chest—the outlook isn't as good. Radiation therapy and chemotherapy, alone or in combination, are the standard treatments. At this stage, the cancer may still be cured.

Patients who already have distant metastases (i.e. stage IV) when they're diagnosed have the worst outlook. Chemotherapy at this stage has been shown to improve survival and the quality of life. Radiation therapy is used as palliative care to treat pain, difficulty breathing (from local metastases to the bone or a major airway), and for brain metastases.

Questions to Ask about Your Treatment

Questions you may want to ask about your overall treatment plan include these:

- What treatment do you recommend? Why?
- What can I do to prepare for treatment?
- Will I be able to drive myself to treatment?
- Can I have a friend or family member with me during treatment?
- How long will the treatment last?
- How will I know the treatment is working?
- What if the treatment is unsuccessful or I get worse during treatment?
- Do you recommend that I participate in a clinical trial? Why or why not?
- If I have questions, whom should I call?

(continued)

Questions you may want to ask about surgery include these:

- Am I a good candidate for surgery? Why or why not?
- What type of surgery will be performed? Why?
- What are the potential benefits of this surgery?
- What are the potential risks and complications of this surgery?
- Will this surgery remove all the cancer?
- Should I have chemotherapy and/or radiation therapy in addition to the surgery?
- What can I do to prepare for surgery?
- How long will I be in the hospital?
- What should I expect in the first few days after surgery?
- How will my pain be managed in the hospital and at home?
- Will I need extra assistance at home after the surgery? Will I need oxygen?
- How soon will I be able to return to my normal activities after the surgery?
- Will I have any permanent restrictions on activity after the surgery?
- If I have questions, whom should I call?

Questions you may want to ask about chemotherapy include these:

- Will I need chemotherapy? Why or why not?
- If I need chemotherapy, what drugs will be used?
- How often will I get the drugs, and for how long?
- What side effects should I expect?

(continued)

- How will my side effects be managed?
- What can I do to prepare for chemotherapy?
- If I have questions, whom should I call?

Questions you may want to ask about radiation include these:

- Will I need radiation therapy? Why or why not?
- How often will I get treatments, and for how long?
- What side effects should I expect?
- How will my side effects be managed?
- What can I do to prepare for radiation therapy?
- If I have questions, whom should I call?

Chapter 5

Treating Small Cell Lung Cancer

S mall cell lung cancer can grow and spread more quickly than non–small cell lung cancer. Whenever possible, treatment needs to begin quickly. The treatment plan may involve some difficult decisions. Take the time to make sure you understand all the options, but don't delay.

Standard Treatment for Small Cell Lung Cancer

An unfortunate fact about small cell lung cancer, one that needs to be stated at the start, is that for most patients, current treatments do not cure the cancer. The main goal of treatment for both limited-stage and extensive-stage SCLC is to prolong survival and maintain the patient's quality of life. With that in mind, treatment for small cell lung cancer is usually helpful and worth doing—the benefits almost always outweigh the drawbacks.

Every patient with SCLC is different, and your treatment will be individualized for you, depending on the stage of your cancer, overall health, and personal preferences. The treatment plan you work out with your health care providers will be different than the treatment someone else with small cell lung cancer might receive.

Standard treatment for small cell lung cancer is based on many years of experience and research. The treatments have become the standards because doctors know they work and they know what to expect. Several types of standard treatment are used for small cell lung cancer:

- **Surgery.** By the time most people are diagnosed, small cell lung cancer has almost always spread to nearby lymph nodes or other parts of the body. Surgery isn't usually appropriate at this point. Occasionally, surgery will be performed to diagnose a lung nodule that then turns out to be small cell carcinoma.

- **Chemotherapy.** In chemotherapy, drugs to stop or slow the growth of the cancer are given. It's called systemic because it reaches all the cells in the body. Because cancer cells grow much faster than most cells in your body, the drugs affect the cancer cells much more than other cells.

- **Radiation therapy.** Radiation therapy uses high-energy x-ray beams or other types of radiation to kill cancer cells or keep them from growing. External radiation therapy uses high-tech machines to deliver a very targeted beam to the cancer, while avoiding the healthy tissue around the cancer.

Treatment of Limited-Stage Small Cell Lung Cancer

The treatment options for limited-stage small cell lung cancer are complex. To decide on your treatment plan, you and your medical team will need to consider your overall health and your personal desires.

Patients with limited-stage SCLC have cancer that hasn't spread that far. It's still only in one lung and in the lymph nodes in the lung, and nearby, and it hasn't spread into other parts of the body.

Combination chemotherapy and external radiation therapy to the chest administered at the same time is the standard treatment for patients who are in relatively good health. This treatment is known as concurrent treatment and combined modality treatment. Patients receive doublet chemotherapy—treatment that combines two drugs. The first is platinum-based drug, either cisplatin or carboplatin. The second is often a drug called etoposide, but a different drug may be used instead, depending on what your medical oncologist feels will work best for you. Most patients receive four to six cycles of the chemotherapy. Each cycle is three weeks; depending on the drugs being used, you will receive treatment on the first day of the cycle and sometimes again a week later, on the eighth day. Chest radiation, also called thoracic radiotherapy (TRTx) sometimes begins along with the first chemotherapy treatment, but it may be delayed for a cycle or two so your doctor can see how well you do on the chemo. The radiation may be given twice daily, a few hours apart, five days a week, for three weeks—a schedule known as accelerated hyperfractionated radiation therapy.

Combined modality treatment for limited-stage SCLC is meant to cure the cancer, but in reality, cure rates are low. The treatment is most effective for prolonging survival and maintaining quality of life.

The side effects of the chemotherapy part include fatigue, nausea and vomiting, and mouth sores. Fortunately, today we have excellent drugs that help prevent and control nausea and vomiting, the two most worrisome side effects. The side effects of radiation include difficulty swallowing (esophagitis), lung inflammation (pneumonitis), and coughing. Medication for these side effects can be very helpful for relieving the symptoms. For many patients, the biggest side effect of combined modality treatment is fatigue, especially during the radiation portion of the treatment. There aren't any drugs for fatigue, but it is manageable just by taking things very easy, getting plenty of sleep, and eating well to keep up your strength. (We'll discuss ways to make treatment as easy as possible in detail in chapter 6.)

For patients who have other lung problems or are ill from other health problems, such as heart failure, standard treatment is modified to make it as safe and effective as possible.

Most patients will have a good response to concurrent treatment. That can mean that the patient goes into complete remission—all evidence of the cancer is gone when the treatment is completed. A partial response—where the tumor shrinks by more than 50 percent—is also considered to be a good response.

Patients who have a good response to concurrent chemoradiotherapy or combination chemotherapy may also later have radiation therapy to the brain to help keep the cancer from spreading (metastasizing) there. We'll discuss brain radiation in more detail later in this chapter.

Treatment of Extensive-Stage Small Cell Lung Cancer

The most commonly used standard treatment for extensive-stage small cell lung cancer is combination chemotherapy, usually using the platinum-based drugs cisplatin or carboplatin, in combination with another drug such as etoposide.

In extensive-stage SCLC, the cancer has usually already spread to other parts of the body, such as the brain, spine, bones, or liver. Chemotherapy alone will often shrink the tumors elsewhere in the body. Radiation therapy may be used at this stage to target a tumor outside the lung that is causing serious symptoms, such as pain.

Treatment of Recurrent Small Cell Lung Cancer

Unfortunately, many patients with small cell lung cancer, even those who respond well to treatment, will relapse. The cancer recurs, sometimes only a few months after treatment. If the relapse happens early (in less than three months) and if the patient is fit enough to tolerate it, then the treatment is usually to try a different type of chemotherapy, often including a drug called topotecan. If the relapse occurs later on, more chemotherapy can be tried, using the same drugs as the first time.

In addition, radiation therapy can be used relieve pain and other symptoms and to improve the quality of life, whether or not the patient is a candidate for additional chemotherapy.

Clinical Trials

If standard treatment isn't working well, or if you're not a good candidate for standard treatment, talk to your doctor about participating in a clinical trial. The purpose of clinical trials is to learn if a new cancer treatment—a new drug or a new type of radiation treatment, for example—is safe and effective and if it might be better than standard treatment. Patients who participate in clinical trials usually receive standard treatment plus an additional drug or a different type of radiation therapy. Some patients may receive a placebo (a harmless substance) instead of the drug being tested, but they will still receive the rest of the standard therapy. By volunteering for a clinical trial, you may be one of the first patients to receive a new treatment that could turn out to be helpful. You'll also be contributing to the ongoing research that is so important for improving cancer treatment. Many of today's standard treatments were developed on the basis of clinical trials.

Because clinical trials are so important for helping move cancer treatment ahead, and because patients often benefit from the treatment, we'll go into them in more detail in chapter 7 on new treatments for lung cancer.

Brain Metastases in Small Cell Lung Cancer

When small cell lung cancer metastasizes beyond the lung, one of the most likely places for it to go is to the brain. Even though the new tumor is in the brain, it's still lung cancer, and the treatment is different than it would be for a tumor that first arises in the brain. There may be more than one metastasis to the brain, and the cancer may be in any part of the brain. Brain metastases are usually diagnosed by a CT scan or MRI; the tumor can show up on the scan before any symptoms appear.

About 18 percent of all patients with extensive-stage disease already have brain metastases when they are first diagnosed. Over the course of their illness, 40 to 60 percent of patients with extensive-stage small cell lung cancer may develop a brain metastasis.

The most common symptom of a brain metastasis is headache. Other symptoms can include nausea, vomiting, and extreme tiredness. Depending on where the tumor is in the brain, it can also cause weakness in an arm or a leg, difficulty walking or speaking, and vision changes. Sometimes patients have seizures. Some patients have alterations in consciousness such as "spaciness," drowsiness, personality changes, mood changes, and memory problems. Brain metastases can also cause a deep coma, leading to death.

Treating lung cancer that has spread to the brain can be challenging. Symptoms such as headache, nausea, and vomiting are caused by swelling of the brain. Steroid drugs that reduce the swelling can often help relieve these symptoms. Sometimes a single tumor in the brain can be removed by surgery, usually followed by radiation therapy to kill any cancerous cells that might remain. Most patients with advanced lung cancer aren't healthy enough for this, however, and it's not recommended even for healthier patients who have more than one tumor.

In most cases, tumors in the brain are treated with radiation therapy to kill the cancer cells. This treatment is known as whole brain radiotherapy (WBRT). Whole brain radiotherapy usually takes two to three weeks of daily treatment, five days a week. The treatments are painless and very short. To make sure you don't move your head during the treatment, a mask, or "shell," is custom-made to fit over your face and head and attach to the radiation table.

Radiotherapy to the brain can cause side effects such as hair loss, nausea and vomiting, and increasing drowsiness over the days as the treatment goes on. Some patients also have memory problems. Hair usually grows back within a few months, and medication taken before each treatment can be very helpful for the nausea and vomiting. The fatigue is unavoidable but usually gets slowly better over a few weeks after treatment is completed. Resting is the only treatment for this side effect. Memory problems from whole brain radiation usually get better once treatment is over.

Preventing Brain Metastases

Some patients are good candidates for radiation treatment to prevent brain metastases. These patients usually have limited-stage disease and have completed combination chemotherapy with good results. Even so, they have about a 60 percent chance of developing at least one metastasis to the brain within the next two to three years. To keep this from happening, the standard treatment is prophylactic (preventive) cranial irradiation (PCI). Studies have shown that for patients with limited-stage disease, PCI can cut the risk of a brain metastasis developing by more than 50 percent, while also extending survival somewhat.

PCI is generally well tolerated, but it can have some side effects, especially for patients over age 60. In the short run, these can include fatigue, hair loss, nausea and vomiting, and memory loss. In the long run, some patients have memory problems, confusion, and difficulty concentrating. The short- and long-term side effects can be distressing, but they're generally considerably better than the side effects of brain metastases. Even so, some patients who are good candidates for PCI decide to take a watchful waiting approach instead. Discuss the pros and cons carefully with your doctor before making your choice

PCI is usually given once per day for five to ten days, but the treatment length can vary. Your radiation oncologist will take your overall health into account when deciding the best approach to PCI for you.

Palliative Treatment for Small Cell Lung Cancer

Sadly, despite all the improvements in diagnosis and treatment doctors have made over the past few decades, the long-term outlook for people with small cell lung cancer is poor. While most people aren't cured, there's still a lot we can do to help keep them comfortable and maintain their quality of life. Palliative care, as this is called, focuses on relieving symptoms such as pain and breathing problems.

Doctors today feel strongly that palliative treatment should be individualized for each patient and that pain control and the patient's comfort should be top priorities. This is such an important topic in treating lung cancer that we'll discuss it in detail in chapter 9.

Questions to Ask about Radiation Therapy

Most patients with limited-stage small cell lung cancer will receive external beam radiation therapy to the chest. Some questions to ask your doctor are these:

- Why do I need radiation therapy?
- How often will I get treatments, and for how long?
- What side effects should I expect?
- How will my side effects be managed?

(continued)

- What can I do to prepare for radiation therapy?
- If I have questions, whom should I call?

If you need radiation to treat metastases to the brain, there are some additional questions to ask:

- Why do I need brain radiation?
- How often will I get treatments, and for how long?
- What side effects should I expect?
- How will my side effects be managed?
- What can I do to prepare for radiation therapy?
- If I have questions, whom should I call?

If your doctor recommends prophylactic brain irradiation (PCI) to prevent brain metastases, some questions to ask are these:

- Why do I need PCI?
- What are the short- and long-term side effects?
- How often will I get treatments, and for how long?
- How will my side effects be managed?
- What can I do to prepare for PCI?
- If I have questions, whom should I call?

Chapter 6

Managing Your Treatment

Going through chemotherapy and radiation therapy or surgery for lung cancer is a real challenge. It can be hard on you, your family, and the people around you, but your treatment team will do everything they can to help you through your treatment. Side effects such as nausea and fatigue can't be avoided, but doctors today have a whole arsenal of medications that help reduce and relieve side effects. In combination with practical steps you can take to help yourself, your treatment side effects can be managed so that you can get through your treatment schedule as comfortably as possible.

Side effects from radiation therapy and chemotherapy vary a lot from patient to patient. Two people with similar cancers receiving similar treatment may have different responses—one person might find fatigue is the biggest problem, while the other has more trouble with nausea. The type of side effects and how mild or severe they are aren't an indication of how well the treatment is working. (The exception is some targeted therapy drugs, as we'll discuss in chapter 7. Their side effects may mean they are working, and fortunately the side effects are mild and easy to manage.) Bad side effects from chemotherapy or radiation simply mean you need to have better medication and care to relieve them.

Because medications today are very effective for treating side effects with few side effects of their own, patients should ask for all the help they need. Doctors agree: no cancer patient should "tough out" side effects or pain when drugs and other steps that help are available.

The side effects of chemotherapy and radiation have different causes, but they're generally treated and prevented in the same way. In this chapter, we'll talk about side effects, treatment, and prevention by symptom and discuss the cause as necessary.

Fatigue

Fatigue—feeling weak and very tired all the time—is a common side effect of both chemotherapy and radiation therapy. The best way to cope is to use some simple strategies to plan around your tiredness:

- Do the activities that are most important to you first, while you still have the energy.

- Listen to your body. If you feel tired, rest or take a short nap; try to sleep eight hours each night.

- Ask others to help you and do less yourself.

- If you can, take time off from your job or work fewer hours.

- Eat well and be sure to drink plenty of fluids (see below for more on this).

- Getting some gentle exercise each day can actually give you more energy. Try a short walk, gentle stretching, yoga, or a short workout on an exercise bike or treadmill.

Fatigue from chemotherapy is usually worse in the days right after treatment and gradually gets better. Fatigue from radiation therapy gets worse as the treatment goes on. After your treatment ends, your energy will gradually return.

Sometimes pain, insomnia, or depression can make fatigue worse. If you're in pain, having trouble sleeping, or feeling depressed and hopeless, talk to your doctor. There's a lot that can be done to help the underlying problems that are contributing to your fatigue. (We'll talk about all three problems in more depth later in this chapter.)

Poor nutrition may also be a factor in fatigue. It's important to eat well during your treatment to help keep up your energy. That can be difficult, especially when you feel nauseous—check the tips we give below for some ideas on how to get good nutrition despite chemo and radiation side effects. Poor nutrition can cause anemia (a shortage of oxygen-carrying red blood cells) from a lack of iron in the diet or from a lack of vitamin B12.

Chemotherapy affects the bone marrow, where your red blood cells are produced. Your bone marrow may not be able to make a normal number of red blood cells, also resulting in anemia. Your red blood cells will gradually return to normal or close to normal once you finish chemotherapy.

Red blood cells carry oxygen to the rest of your body, and when you don't have enough of them to get oxygen to all your cells, you can start to feel very fatigued. Symptoms of severe anemia include feeling dizzy or faint, being short of breath, feeling unusually weak and very tired, and having a rapid heartbeat. Call your doctor at once if you notice any of these symptoms.

If your fatigue is from severe anemia caused by chemotherapy, a blood transfusion can increase your red blood cell count. As an alternative, your doctor may suggest giving you shots of a drug called epoetin alfa (Epogen or Procrit) or darbepoetin (Aranesp). The drugs stimulate your bone marrow to produce more red blood cells, just as erythropoietin, a substance produced by your kidneys naturally does. These drugs can be very helpful and are usually very safe to use. They can also have some serious side effects. The shots can make your body ache, they may give you a headache or diarrhea, and they may cause high blood pressure. More seriously, they can cause life-threatening blood clots, especially when they're given to people who have anemia but are no longer in chemotherapy. They can also increase your risk for heart problems, including heart attack, stroke, and heart failure.

When you discuss epoetin alfa or darbepoetin treatment with your doctor, bear the possible risks in mind. Some questions to ask include the following:

- Is this drug safe for me?
- Will it help with my fatigue?

- Are the side effects worth the risk?
- Would a transfusion be safer or better for me?

Discuss your fatigue issues with your treatment team and be sure to speak up if your fatigue starts to interfere with your activities of daily living or suddenly gets worse.

Nausea and Vomiting

One of the most common side effects of chemotherapy and radiation for lung cancer is nausea and sometimes vomiting. Because this a very common side effect of almost any treatment for any cancer, your treatment team has a lot of experience in helping patients deal with it. Today many very effective drugs can help keep treatment-related nausea and vomiting to a minimum. The medical term for vomiting or throwing up is *emesis,* so these drugs are known as antiemetic agents.

Cisplatin, the most widely used drug for lung cancer, often causes nausea. Etoposide, another widely used drug, has a lower risk but can also cause nausea. Prevention is the best way to manage the nausea from these drugs. Your doctor will probably prescribe antinausea medication for you to take before, during, and after the days when you have a chemotherapy treatment. Take the drugs on schedule, even if you don't feel nauseous—they work best as prevention and may not help as much if you wait to take them until you feel sick to your stomach.

Radiation to the chest is less likely to cause nausea and vomiting, but the risk is still there. Radiation to the brain can also cause nausea and vomiting. In most cases, the symptoms happen soon after treatment, usually within 30 minutes to several hours. Your doctor will probably prescribe an antinausea drug for you to take before each treatment.

Some people experience anticipatory nausea. This usually happens after you've already had several chemotherapy or radiation treatments. The smells, sights, and sounds of the treatment room trigger nausea even before the treatment begins. For many patients, relaxation techniques or distraction, such as listening to music, watching a video, or playing a video game, help prevent anticipatory nausea.

Despite all the antinausea drugs, you may still end up vomiting. Usually the vomiting will stop once your stomach is empty. Aside from the unpleasantness of it, frequent vomiting can cause dehydration—a dangerous loss of fluids in the body. Watch for symptoms such as dry mouth, sticky saliva, reduced urine output, or urine that is dark yellow. Call your doctor or go to the emergency room if you are vomiting often and show signs of dehydration. You may need an intravenous drug to stop the vomiting and intravenous fluids to treat the dehydration.

If you have uncontrolled vomiting, your doctor may want to try a different antinausea drug. There are many good options. If one drug isn't working well for you, don't hesitate to tell your care team and ask to try a different one or add a new drug. Sometimes it takes a combination of two or more drugs to give you full relief. One drawback to some antinausea drugs is that they can cause constipation. If the drug is working well for you otherwise, this side effect can be easily managed. If the drug isn't working that well and is also making you constipated, discuss trying something else with your doctor.

Self-Help for Nausea and Vomiting

Many effective steps can be taken at home to help prevent and relieve nausea and vomiting. The most important is to take the antinausea drugs your doctor has prescribed, even if you don't feel sick at the moment.

Some other self-help steps include the following:

- Drink frequently in small amounts. Cool liquids such as plain water; plain tea; clear fruit juices like apple, cranberry, or grape juice; and flat ginger ale are all good choices. If you've been throwing up a lot, oral rehydration drinks, such as Pedialyte, can help restore lost fluids and make you feel better. Avoid fizzy drinks and alcohol.

- Eat small meals throughout the day instead of three larger meals. Don't force yourself to eat, but if you do feel hungry, eat something.

- If you feel nauseous when you get up in the morning, try nibbling on plain toast, crackers, dry breakfast cereal, pretzels, and other bland, dry foods.

- Avoid fatty, spicy, fried, and very sweet foods.

- For main meals, stick to bland foods such as baked chicken without the skin, oatmeal, cream of rice or cream of wheat cereal, plain pasta or noodles, boiled potatoes without the skin, and white rice. Bananas; canned fruit such as applesauce, peaches, and pears; JELL-O; ice pops; and plain yogurt are all good snacks.

- Strong food smells can trigger nausea. Cold or room temperature foods can help with this. Stay out of the kitchen while food is being cooked.

- Avoid lying flat for at least two hours after a meal.

- Suck on sugar-free mints or hard candies or chew sugar-free gum if you feel nauseous.

- If you find you get nauseous during treatment, avoid eating for a few hours before. Some people feel better if they eat a small meal before treatment, but others feel better if they avoid eating or drinking. Be guided by your own experience and how you feel.

- Slow, deep breathing or getting some fresh air can help control an attack of nausea. So does distraction. Watch TV, talk with a friend, listen to music, do something with your hands—anything that takes your mind off your stomach will help.

- Ginger, a traditional nausea remedy, may help relieve nausea from chemotherapy. Try swallowing a quarter teaspoon of chopped fresh ginger or drinking a cup of tea made from half a teaspoon of chopped fresh ginger before treatment. Capsules containing dried ginger are available at health food stores. If you decide to try ginger for nausea, be sure to tell your doctor.

While you're in treatment, you will probably have to limit alcoholic drinks or even avoid them completely. Discuss alcohol use with your doctor.

Loss of Appetite and Difficulty Eating

Losing your appetite is another very common side effect of treatment for lung cancer. It's generally due to nausea from chemotherapy, and many of the same self-help techniques discussed above can help. In addition, try these ideas to make sure you get enough calories each day to keep up your strength:

- Eat several small meals a day and snack whenever you feel hungry.

- If you do feel hungry, don't limit how much you eat.

- For meals, try plain baked or broiled chicken, eggs, cottage cheese, and fish. Liquid meal replacements are good if you can't face a solid meal.

- Eat nutritious snacks that are high in calories. Good snack choices include cereal, pudding, nuts, muffins, milkshakes and smoothies, ice cream, and granola bars. Keep your favorites on hand for easy snacking.

- Increase the calories and nutrition in your meals by adding gravy, sauce, butter, cheese, peanut butter, nuts, or cream to your food—unless you know these make you nauseated.

- If you don't feel up to solid foods, try to drink a lot of fluids. Juices, soups, instant breakfast drinks, smoothies and milkshakes, and whole milk are all good choices.

- Drink liquids between meals, not with meals. Drinking during the meal can make you feel full too quickly.

- Try to get some light exercise, such as short walk, before meals to stimulate your appetite.
- Tell your doctor or nurse if you lose weight.

Cisplatin often gives you a metallic or bitter taste in your mouth, which can affect how your food tastes. To maintain good nutrition while you're getting cisplatin, eat the foods that do still taste good to you—experiment a bit to discover which those are. Cold or frozen foods may taste better than hot foods. Sucking on sugar-free mints or candies or chewing sugar-free gum can help mask the metallic taste. The taste in your mouth usually goes away a few days after treatment.

Radiation therapy usually causes weight loss of about one to two pounds a week. This is normal, in part because you may not feel very hungry and in part because your body is burning a lot of calories to repair the damage from the radiation. To keep from losing too much weight and adding to your fatigue, try to eat well, using the suggestions above.

Eating well during treatment is important to help you stay strong. If your appetite loss is severe or you lose more weight than expected, your doctor may want you to see a registered dietitian to help you find ways to maintain good nutrition.

Mouth Problems

Chemotherapy can cause painful mouth sores (stomatitis) or inflammation of the mouth and throat (mucositis), which make it difficult to eat even though you're hungry. Your doctor can prescribe medication that will help. To be sure you're getting good nutrition, try these self-help steps as well:

- Drink cold liquids and eat frozen juice pops or ice pops.

- Eat soft, wet foods that are easy to swallow, such as pudding, custard, JELL-O, and ice cream. Cooked cereals, scrambled eggs, and mashed potatoes are other good choices.

- Soften foods with gravy or sauce.

- Mash or blend foods.

- Drink from a straw.

- Avoid acidic foods, such as oranges and tomatoes.

- Eat cool or cold foods if hot foods are painful.

- Don't drink alcohol.

- Avoid spicy, salty, acidic, and crunchy or hard foods.

To help relieve pain from mouth sores, rinse your mouth with a baking soda mix every few hours during the day. To make the rinse, mix together one cup warm water, one-fourth teaspoon baking soda, and one-eighth teaspoon salt. Stir until the salt dissolves, then take small sips, swish them around in your mouth, and spit them out.

Call your doctor if you notice white spots or a white coating inside your mouth or on your tongue. The spots may resemble cottage cheese. You may have oral thrush, a fungal infection that is not uncommon in patients having chemotherapy. Thrush is treated with an antifungal medication, which usually helps quickly.

Because your treatment will lower your resistance to infection, avoid doing any dental work during this time. If possible, visit your dentist for a checkup, cleaning, and any work that needs to be done at least two weeks before you start treatment.

Good dental care is important while you are in treatment. Brush your teeth gently after each meal and before you go to bed. Use a very soft toothbrush and a toothpaste that contains fluoride and baking soda. Floss very gently. Avoid mouthwashes. If you have dentures, try not to wear them—during this time they can cause sores on the gums and inside of the mouth.

Swallowing Problems

Radiation therapy to the chest can make it difficult or painful for you to swallow, a condition called dysphagia. Your doctor can prescribe medicine to help reduce inflammation and pain. Swallowing problems may make you gag or choke on your food. To avoid this and continue to get good nutrition while you're receiving radiation therapy, follow the self-help steps for mouth sores described above. In addition, sit upright while you're eating or drinking. Take small bites or sips. Thicker liquids are easier to swallow, so try thickening liquids by adding tapioca, baby rice cereal, or a commercial thickening agent.

Your doctor may want you to see a speech therapist, who can help you learn ways to swallow better, and a registered dietitian, who can help you learn how to eat nutritiously while you have dysphagia.

Pain

Surgery for lung cancer can leave you feeling very sore and in pain for a long time afterward. While you're doing chemotherapy and radiation, the surgery pain may still be with you. In addition, the treatments can cause muscle and bone aches, pain from neuropathy (see below for more on that), and pain from skin irritation due to radiation. You may also have pain because the cancer has spread to your bones or because the tumor is pressing on nerves.

It's just as important to treat pain as it is to treat any other problem caused by your treatment. Your treatment team members will routinely ask you about your pain. Give them an honest answer. Don't feel you need to minimize your discomfort or that asking for pain relief is a sign of weakness.

Some patients worry about becoming addicted to pain medication. This is rarely a problem for cancer patients because the drugs are necessary—you're not taking them recreationally. When you're feeling better and don't need them as much or at all, you'll almost certainly be able to taper off the drugs easily and not want them anymore. While you're taking pain meds, your body will gradually develop a tolerance for them, and you may need to increase the dose or change the way you take the drug. Tolerance is normal—it isn't addiction—and you will be able to cut back as your pain improves.

Pain can also be treated by other steps in addition to narcotic drugs. Radiation can help relieve pain from bone metastases, nerve blocks can help for pain following lung cancer surgery, and other drugs can help with the pain from neuropathy. If you're having trouble getting your pain under control, ask for a referral to doctor who's a specialist in pain management. (We'll talk more about treating pain with drugs and other methods in chapter 9.)

Talking to Your Doctor about Pain

If you're in pain, communicating clearly with your doctor is important to make sure you get full relief. Make some notes to yourself about the pain:

- On a scale of 1 to 10, where 1 is no pain at all and 10 is the worst pain you can imagine, how would you rate your pain?

- Is it a new pain?

- Where is the pain? Does it move from one place to another?

- How does the pain feel? Is it a dull ache, a sharp stabbing sensation, a burning feeling?

- Does the painful area feel numb, tingly, or weak?

- Is the pain keeping your from your normal daily activities?

- What activities or conditions make the pain worse? What helps?

Tell your doctor about any pain medications you are already taking, including over-the-counter medications such as acetaminophen (Tylenol) or ibuprofen (Advil).

Taking your pain medicine the right way helps it work much better. Discuss what you need to do to get good pain relief from your medicine with your doctor or nurse:

- Be sure to take the recommended amount of pain medicine, not too little or too much.

- Take your pain medicine on the schedule your doctor recommends. If you delay or skip your dose, the drug may not work as well when you finally do take it.

- Tell your doctor or nurse if the medicine isn't helping the pain, is helping less than it used to, isn't working as quickly, or is wearing off sooner.

- Tell your doctor or nurse if you have any new pain or if you are getting pain that comes on quickly (breakthrough pain).

- If you want to stop taking your pain medicine or reduce the dose, discuss it with your doctor first.

Side effects from pain medications include nausea, sleepiness, and constipation. Discuss your side effects with your doctor or nurse for advice on managing them or switching to a different drug.

Self-Help for Pain

Self-help steps can do a lot to relieve pain, but they're no substitute for medication if you need it. Try these ideas to reduce pain:

- Apply gentle heat from a heating pad to aching muscles and joints. Talk to your doctor or nurse first to be sure putting heat on the area is safe for you.

- Ice packs can sometimes be helpful for an area that's sore. Wrap the ice pack in a towel; don't apply it directly to the skin. Talk to your doctor or nurse first to be sure putting ice on the area is safe for you.

- Sucking on chipped ice or a Popsicle can help with the pain from mouth sores.

- Distraction is often very helpful for reducing pain. Watch a funny movie, read a mystery novel, listen to music, talk with friends—anything that takes your mind off the pain will help.

- Mild exercise, such as a short walk, often helps reduce pain.

- Relaxation techniques, such as guided imagery and meditation, can help a lot with pain.

- Gentle massage from a professional masseuse trained in treating cancer patients can help you relax and feel less pain.

- Acupuncture helps some people.

When cancer spreads to the bones and some other organs, it can be very painful. The treatment for severe pain from advanced cancer is a complicated subject. We'll discuss it in depth in chapter 9.

Coughing

Lung cancer patients may have a chronic cough from before they were diagnosed, or they may develop one from the radiation treatment or because the cancer has spread. An old cough may be related to earlier treatment for lung cancer, or it may come from underlying lung disease, such as emphysema. It may even be unrelated to lung problems—sometimes coughing is caused by postnasal drip or by gastroesophageal reflux disease (GERD).

A new cough is more worrisome—call your doctor. It may be a sign of infection, which can be serious, especially while you're doing chemotherapy. A new cough could be caused by the treatment itself—radiation to the chest can cause coughing. It might also be caused by the tumor blocking or pressing on an airway. Any new cough needs to evaluated by your doctor, especially if you cough up blood (hemoptysis).

Coughing can be painful and can keep you from sleeping. Sometimes nonprescription cough medicines can help with an old cough; discuss these with your doctor before you try them. Your doctor may prescribe a narcotic medicine to help relieve an old cough. Treatment of a new cough depends on the underlying cause. Don't use cough medicine for a new cough unless your doctor tells you to.

Avoiding Infection

White blood cells, which protect your body from infection, are made in the bone marrow. Chemotherapy affects the bone marrow and keeps it from making white blood cells. When your overall white blood cell (WBC) count is low, you also have an abnormally low level of neutrophils, a type of white blood cell that's your body's primary defense against bacteria. This condition is called neutropenia. It makes you very vulnerable to getting an infection, and if you do get one, your body will have a hard time fighting it off. A serious infection can not only make you sick and miserable, it can cause dose reductions or delays in your treatment.

Avoiding infection is crucial during this time. You may be given an antibiotic along with your chemotherapy to help prevent infection. In addition, the self-help steps below are extremely important to follow, even if they make you seem a little obsessive or antisocial. It's far better to be too cautious than to risk an infection.

Hand Washing

The single most important step you can take to protect yourself from infection is to wash your hands frequently. Always wash your hands well before you cook or eat, after you use the bathroom, and after being in a public place such as the supermarket.

Wash your hands thoroughly—for at least 20 seconds—using soap and water. Ask the people around you to wash their hands well, too. If soap and water aren't available, use an alcohol-based hand sanitizer, such as PURELL.

Take a daily shower, using a mild soap. Use a gentle, fragrance-free skin lotion to moisturize.

Avoiding Germs

Stay away from people who are sick or who have a cold during your treatment, even if this means skipping a visit to or from someone you care about. Also stay away from people (usually children) who have just had a vaccine for chicken pox, polio, or measles. Ask your doctor about getting a flu shot and the shingles (*Herpes zoster*) vaccine before you start your treatment.

If you can, avoid crowds and public places such as movie theaters.

Avoid food-borne illnesses, such as salmonella, by washing raw fruits and vegetables thoroughly. Wash your hands after you handle raw meat; cook all meat thoroughly. Skip raw foods such as sushi.

Have someone else clean up after your pet, especially the cat litter box.

Brush your teeth carefully with a soft toothbrush.

Avoid cuts, scrapes, and anything else that breaks the skin. Wear gloves when doing dishes, housework, and gardening. Use an electric shaver, not a razor. Trim your fingernails carefully; consider having a podiatrist (foot specialist) cut your toenails.

Danger Signs

Even a minor infection can become serious when your white blood cell count is low. You're particularly vulnerable to bacterial infections that attack your mouth, skin, urinary tract, lungs, rectum, and genital area. *Call your doctor at once or go to the emergency room if you have any of these symptoms during your treatment:*

- A fever of 100.5 degrees Fahrenheit (38 degrees Celsius) or higher
- Chills or sweating
- A new cough, shortness of breath, or sore throat
- Pain or burning when you urinate or frequent urination; urine that is bloody, cloudy, or has a bad odor
- Diarrhea or sores around the anus
- Ear pain
- Stiff or sore neck
- Headache or bad sinus pain
- A new skin rash
- Sores or a white coating in your mouth or on your tongue
- Swelling or redness anywhere on your body, especially around a cut or other wound or around the catheter or port used to give your chemotherapy

Don't hesitate to call your doctor if you have infection symptoms, especially if you have a fever. Prompt treatment with antibiotics or an antifungal drug is very important for stopping the infection quickly. You may need to be hospitalized to receive intravenous antibiotics.

Treating Neutropenia

If your white blood cell count drops dangerously low, your doctor may recommend shots of white blood cell growth factors, also known as granulocyte colony-stimulating factors

(G-CSFs). These drugs are proteins that help the body produce white blood cells. The shot is usually given 24 hours after a chemotherapy treatment. Commonly used G-CSFs include filgrastim (Neupogen), sargramostim (Leukine), and pegfilgrastim (Neulasta).

While these drugs can lower your risk of serious infection, they also have side effects, including aching bones and joints, low-grade fever, and a general sense of feeling unwell (malaise). Also, if you're receiving chemotherapy and radiation therapy at the same time, treatment with G-CSF is not recommended. In general, the shots are recommended if your risk of developing a fever with neutropenia is greater than 20 percent. That's a complex decision—discuss G-CSF treatment with your doctor to decide if the shots are appropriate for you. If these drugs aren't right for you, it may be necessary to lower your next dose of chemotherapy.

Bleeding

Your bone marrow also produces platelets (thrombocytes), tiny particles that travel in your bloodstream and help your blood clot if you have a cut or bruise. Chemotherapy and radiation therapy lower your production of platelets, just as they lower your production of red and white blood cells. When you have thrombocytopenia—the medical term for abnormally low platelets—you can develop bleeding problems because you don't have enough platelets for your blood to clot normally.

Avoiding cuts, scrapes, and bruises is important while your platelet count is low. Follow these self-help steps:

- Use an electric shaver, not a razor.

- Be careful when using knives, scissors, nail clippers, tools, and other sharp objects.

- Protect your feet by wearing shoes or slippers all the time.

- Use a very soft toothbrush. Avoid dental floss and toothpicks.

- Blow your nose very gently.

- Don't play contact sports.

- Use pads, not tampons.

Talk to your doctor before taking any vitamins, supplements, or over-the-counter medications such as aspirin or ibuprofen (Advil). Aspirin can affect your platelets, and some supplements, such as ginkgo biloba, can thin your blood and make bleeding problems worse.

When to Call the Doctor

Bleeding problems can be serious and need immediate attention. Call your doctor at once or go to the emergency room if you notice any of the following:

- Red, pinpoint spots on the skin

- Bruises even though you haven't banged into anything

- Blood or a pink tinge in your urine

- Bowel movements that look black or bloody

- Vomit that looks like coffee grounds

- Bleeding from the mouth or nose
- Bleeding from the vagina when you are not having your period
- Bad headaches, vision changes, or feeling very confused or sleepy

If you start to bleed from a cut, press down firmly on the area with a clean cloth. Keep pressing until the bleeding stops. If it doesn't stop within a few minutes, call your doctor or go to the emergency room. If you bruise yourself, put ice on the area for about 20 minutes.

Your doctor may recommend a platelet transfusion or possibly a delay in your next treatment if your platelet count falls too low. Transfusion can be done in the doctor's office unless other problems require hospitalization.

Peripheral Neuropathy

Cisplatin, the drug used most commonly used to treat lung cancer, can cause a nerve problem called peripheral neuropathy. When you have peripheral neuropathy, you usually have a numb, tingling, burning, or weak feeling in your hands or feet. The tingling can be painful—it's often described as a sharp cutting sensation or feeling like you're being stuck with a needle. Peripheral neuropathy can also cause movement problems, such as falling, losing your balance, shaking or trembling muscles, and trouble holding or picking up things. It can even become hard to button your shirt or tie your shoelaces.

Peripheral neuropathy can get worse as your treatment continues. For mild neuropathy, over-the-counter drugs such as aspirin or ibuprofen (Advil) can help. Ice packs can also help hand and foot discomfort. To relieve more severe neuropathy, your doctor may prescribe stronger medications. Peripheral neuropathy usually slowly gets better after you stop chemotherapy, but you may have some long-term effects.

Because your feet and hands may be numb and your sense of balance may be affected, it's important to take steps at home to avoid injury:

- Prevent falls by removing throw rugs and making sure electrical wires and other obstacles, such as footstools, are out of the way.
- Put up grab rails in the bathroom.
- Put bathmats in the shower and tub.
- Wear sturdy shoes that fit well. Avoid wearing loose-fitting slippers and don't go barefoot.
- Use a cane or walker if necessary.
- Use pot holders in the kitchen to avoid burns.
- Be sure the water in the shower or tub isn't too hot before you step in. Ask someone else to check if possible.
- Wear gloves when you are doing housework, gardening, or working outside.
- Check your feet for cuts or other skin breaks every day.
- Ask for help with buttoning clothes, opening jars, and anything else that has become difficult for you.

- Don't drive if you can't feel the pedals or hold the steering wheel well.

Sometimes physical therapy can be helpful for relieving neuropathy pain and learning how to do things differently to work around numbness, balance problems, and so on. If you need a cane or walker, a physical therapist can teach you the right way to use them. Ask your doctor if seeing a physical therapist is a good idea for you.

Skin Problems

External radiation can irritate the skin of the irradiated area. The skin often gets red and peels, much like when you get a bad sunburn. The damage usually starts after one or two weeks of treatment and starts to get better as soon as treatment stops. The skin is usually back to normal within a few weeks. During this time, treat your skin gently. Don't put any skin products, such as perfume, powders, lotions, ointments, or cosmetics, on the affected area, especially if they contain alcohol. (Your doctor may recommend an ointment that can help soothe the area.) Use a mild soap and lukewarm water, and don't rub, scrub, or scratch the area. Wear loose clothing over the treated area and avoid exposing it to the sun. You'll need to avoid sunlight and tanning beds on the treated area for a year after completing treatment.

Sleeping Problems

Many people with cancer have trouble sleeping, at least some of the time. In fact, studies have shown that more than half of all people with advanced cancer experience insomnia. Coping with a cancer diagnosis and then treatment is extremely stressful. It's not surprising that many patients have insomnia, bad dreams, and other sleep problems. On top of the fatigue that goes with cancer treatment, sleeping problems can leave you feeling exhausted, depressed, anxious, and irritable. Lack of sleep can also slow down your healing from surgery and your recovery from treatment.

The first step in treating your sleep problems is to deal with underlying causes, such as pain or nausea. As explained earlier in this chapter, very effective medications can help with these—don't hesitate to discuss them with your doctor. For lung cancer patients, shortness of breath, which can become worse when you lie down, can keep you from getting a restful night's sleep. If this is a problem for you, discuss it with your doctor—you may need breathing medications or extra oxygen to help. (We'll talk more about treating shortness of breath in chapter 9.)

Some medications, such as decongestants, some antidepressants, and some tobacco-cessation products, can affect your sleep. If you think one of the drugs you're taking is keeping you from sleeping, tell your doctor. You may be able to switch to a different drug that won't keep you up. Your doctor may prescribe sleeping pills, but these are usually effective only for short-term use. If you're also taking pain medications or some other drugs, sleeping pills might not be safe.

Coping with Chemobrain

Cancer treatment is stressful. It also involves a lot of different drugs, often including powerful drugs to treat pain. Not surprisingly, between the stress and the drugs, during treatment many patients feel "foggy," find it hard to concentrate, and have trouble remembering things, a condition informally known as chemobrain. To cope with chemobrain, put important dates on your calendar, make lists, and write notes to yourself. To keep track of your medications, use a pillbox or a calendar. If you need to do something that requires concentration, such as paying bills or filling out paperwork, do it at the time of day you feel best. And if you need extra help, ask a family member or friend. Chemobrain and feeling foggy usually improve over time once you finish treatment.

Depression and anxiety are very normal emotions to experience when you have cancer. These feelings can be very distressing and can keep you up at night. Medications to help you deal with anxiety and depression can be very helpful for some people—ask your doctor if they are appropriate for you.

Whether or not you take medication, relaxation techniques, such as deep breathing and guided imagery, are very useful for helping you cope. Participating in a cancer support group can also be very helpful. The support group is a safe place to express your emotions to people who truly understand what you're going through. Cognitive behavioral therapy (CBT), which uses short, focused sessions to help with specific problems, such as depression, can also be very helpful.

Your oncologist, your social worker, or the patient services department of your local hospital can help you find a cancer support group. Some hospitals keep referral lists for experienced therapists who can teach you relaxation techniques and CBT. Useful videos and books on relaxation techniques are inexpensive and easy to find. (Check the resources listed in appendix B for more information.) No one solution works for everyone—what works to help one person sleep better may not work for you. Keep trying until you find a coping choice that works for you.

Questions to Ask about Managing Your Treatment

- What sorts of problems should I call you about?
- What problems are medical emergencies? When should I go to the hospital?
- What over-the-counter medicines are safe for me to take?
- Do I need to take vitamins?
- What herbal remedies and dietary supplements are not safe for me?
- Do I need a referral to a registered dietitian?
- What should I do if the antinausea medicine isn't working?
- What can I do about fatigue?
- What should I do if the pain medicine isn't working?
- What should I do about shortness of breath?
- Should I see a pain management specialist?
- Should I see a physical therapist?

Chapter 7

Advances in the Evaluation and Management of Lung Cancer

Ongoing research has led to some very promising advances in the evaluation and management of lung cancer. Major advances in prevention, diagnosis, staging, and treatment have occurred in the past decade. Even more exciting progress in these areas is expected to occur over the next decade. The present and the future hold much hope for people with lung cancer.

Prevention

Strict laws banning smoking in public places, such as restaurants, bars, sporting events, and schools, have been in place in most states for a number of years. In 2009, a new law that gives the FDA authority to regulate nicotine, the addictive drug in tobacco, was enacted. The law also strictly regulates other aspects of the tobacco industry, including marketing to young people to entice them to smoke. These laws have helped reduce the number of smokers overall and have reduced the number of young people who become new smokers. They have done a great deal to prevent lung cancer in the future.

In addition to nicotine replacement therapies, prescription drugs that can help you stop smoking, such as Zyban, Wellbutrin (bupropion), or Chantix (varenicline), are now available.

Advances in Imaging

PET imaging, as we described in chapter 2, has been a major advance in lung cancer diagnosis and staging. This test is very helpful for diagnosing lung nodules and for staging lung cancer within the chest and throughout the body.

Advances in Bronchoscopy

Traditional bronchoscopy using a standard bronchoscope is tricky. It's hard to reach small nodules with the bronchoscope, because they're deep within the lungs, beyond where the camera on the end of the bronchoscope can see. Because the main airways branch into many thousands of ever-smaller airways, it's also hard to know if the bronchoscope is following the correct branch of the lung to reach the nodule. If we can't reach the nodule with the bronchoscope to do a biopsy, a more invasive surgical method may have to be used—and that can be a problem for people with poor lung function.

A new technique called electromagnetic navigation bronchoscopy lets us locate and biopsy lung nodules and lymph nodes that are difficult or impossible to reach with traditional bronchoscopy. The system is similar to the GPS technology now in widespread use for navigation throughout the world. The electromagnetic navigation bronchoscopy equipment creates a three-dimensional virtual "road map" of your lungs, based on a CT scan. The doctor uses special bronchoscopy equipment to navigate through your lungs to reach the targeted area.

Endobronchial ultrasound is another new technique that lets us see the lymph nodes that sit just outside the airways. Instead of blindly sticking a biopsy needle into the lymph nodes, we can now see the needle as it goes in and be sure it's going into the right place. That helps us get better biopsy samples from the lymph nodes in the chest, which in turn makes for staging the lung cancer more accurately and less invasively. The same technique works for seeing and doing a biopsy on small lung nodules.

Targeted Therapies

Targeted therapies—drugs that target only the cells within a tumor—are an exciting new development in treating lung cancer. These new drugs have significantly improved the outlook for many people with lung cancer, even those patients who haven't responded well to other treatments.

Research into the basic biology of cancer cells has given us a much better understanding of how these cells grow, survive chemotherapy and radiation, and manage to spread to other parts of the body. By blocking or modifying some of the basic biological processes that have gone wrong in cancer cells, the new targeted therapies can stop uncontrolled cell growth, block new blood vessels from forming to feed the tumor, and make cancer cells die off. These drugs act much more on the cancer cells than on other growing cells, so they maximize the benefit of treatment while minimizing harm to noncancerous cells.

Today, most doctors think that targeted therapies work best when they're used to treat advanced lung cancer alongside standard chemotherapy with platinum-based drugs, but in some cases, the targeted therapy alone or in combination with another targeted drug can be effective. We're still learning about the best ways to use these drugs and which patients are most likely to benefit from them. In addition, some promising new drugs are in various phases of clinical trials and may become available in the near future.

The targeted therapies currently in use attack two different biologic processes within cancer cells. In both, the drugs block part of the process from happening, which in turn keeps cancer cells from dividing or kills the cancer cells.

Epidermal Growth Factor Receptor Inhibitors

A protein called epidermal growth factor is crucial for making cancer cells divide and grow. Epidermal growth factor binds with special receptors on the surface of a cancer cell and then, in a complex process, stimulates the cell to grow and divide. Drugs that block this process are called epidermal growth factor receptor inhibitors, or EGFR inhibitors for short. Three drugs, erlotinib (Tarceva), cetuximab (Erbitux), and gefitinib (Iressa), are now being used or studied for treating advanced non–small cell lung cancer.

EGFR inhibitors have been studied as frontline therapy in combination with standard chemotherapy for people with advanced NSCLC, as second-line therapy alone or in combination with standard treatment for patients with lung cancer that progressed despite standard first-line chemotherapy, and in combination with other targeted therapies. There studies have generated both tremendous hope and disappointment.

In general, we have learned that this class of medication can lead to dramatic responses in a small portion of lung cancer patients. This group includes women, never-smokers, patients with adenocarcinoma of the lung, and people of Asian decent. Patients whose tumors have particular kinds of mutations in the EGFRs are also likely to have a good response. For some of these patients, the response to the drug can be dramatic, shrinking the tumors and extending life expectancy. For other groups of people with lung cancer, the amount of benefit from this class of medication is less clear.

Some large medical centers now do genetic testing to see if the patient is likely to benefit from an EGFR-inhibiting drug. The tests look for EGFR mutations in the tumor and at the number of copies of some genes to determine in advance who will respond. Gene testing for EGFR response has value now and will doubtless have greater value in the future, but in most cases, the clinical characteristics of the patient are enough to tell us that he or she will probably have a good response.

Skin reactions are very common with EGFR drugs. The most troublesome symptom is an acnelike rash with pimples and red bumps on the face, neck, and upper chest and back. The rash can be very tender and itchy, to the point of interfering with activities of daily living and keeping you from sleeping. The rash can be managed with prescription creams and usually gets better after you've been taking the drug for a while. Diarrhea is the next most common side effect. Other reported side effects include hair loss, fatigue, nail problems,

The Cost of Targeted Therapies

Targeted therapy drugs are extremely expensive. A month of treatment with just one drug can cost between $7,500 and $10,000; combined treatment with two drugs would be even more expensive. Health insurance may cover some or all of the cost, but the uncovered portion and copays can still run into the thousands. The drug manufacturers have special patient-assistance programs for those who have trouble paying for the treatment. If the cost of the treatment is a problem for you or if your insurer is unwilling to pay, talk to your doctor to see what can be done. We hope that in the future, as evidence mounts about their proper use, coverage will expand and the cost will go down.

fingertip fissures, and lung inflammation. One significant advantage of the EGFR drugs is that they can often be taken at home as a pill. Patients don't need to travel to the oncology office for IV treatment.

Angiogenesis Inhibitors

A tumor needs a blood supply to bring it the oxygen and nutrients that let it survive and grow. One hallmark of cancer is that the tumor builds new blood vessels to nourish itself. If the blood supply is cut off, the tumor usually shrinks and becomes inactive. What if there were a way to stop the tumor from making new blood vessels? That's what angiogenesis inhibitor drugs do. (*Angiogenesis* is the scientific term for the growth of new blood vessels.) If there's no angiogenesis, the tumor starves.

An angiogenesis inhibitor called bevacizumab (Avastin) has been approved by the FDA as first-line treatment for non-squamous non–small cell lung cancer in combination with standard chemotherapy. This drug is a vascular endothelial growth factor (VEGF) inhibitor. Blocking this growth factor helps to prevent angiogenesis. The combination of chemotherapy and bevacizumab has been shown to help selected patients have a longer period of progression-free survival and help prolong overall survival.

The decision to try bevacizumab as part of your therapy will depend on a number of factors, including the type and stage of your cancer and your overall health. If bevacizumab is appropriate for you, it will be given intravenously along with your chemotherapy. Because bevacizumab and other vascular endothelial growth factor (VEGF) inhibitors prevent new blood vessel growth, they can cause bleeding in the lungs. Therefore, they are not suggested for use in people at high risk for bleeding in the lungs, such as many patients with squamous cell non–small cell lung cancer. Other side effects can usually be easily managed.

Other angiogenesis inhibitor drugs, such as sunitinib (Sutent) and sorafenib (Nexavar), are approved for other cancers and are being looked at for lung cancer as well. This area of research holds great promise for all cancer patients.

Video-Assisted Thoracic Surgery

In some medical centers, lung surgeons are using video-assisted thoracic surgery (VATS) to remove lung tumors. This procedure is less invasive than standard open surgery. To perform the operation, a thin tube with a tiny video camera on the end is put into the chest cavity through a small hole in the chest wall. One or more additional long, thin tools are inserted into the chest through small holes in the chest wall. The surgeon uses the video camera to see inside the chest and the other instruments to remove the lobe.

VATS uses smaller incisions, which means less pain and a faster recovery for the patient. The technique may not be useful for all lung cancer resections, however. VATS is a fairly new technique. It's not in widespread use yet, because the equipment is complicated and expensive and surgeons need to be thoroughly trained in how to use it. If your doctor recommends a lobectomy, ask if VATS surgery is possible and available to you. You may need to travel to a major medical center to find a surgeon who is skilled in the technique.

Radiosurgery

Radiosurgery uses high-tech radiation systems to attack tumors in the lung and metastases to the brain—it's not really surgery in the traditional sense. This technology was initially developed to treat brain tumors, so clearly the radiation beams can be very accurately targeted at the tumor. The more technically correct name for radiosurgery applied to the lung is stereotactic body radiotherapy (SBRT). The advantage of SBRT over conventional external beam radiation is that the equipment can deliver high doses of radiation to the tumor. The advanced targeting used in SBRT means less radiation reaches normal tissues. SBRT treatment is over more quickly. Instead of weeks of daily treatment, SBRT for lung cancer usually takes three to five treatments. With some types of stereotactic radiation equipment, patients wear a special vest with sensors on it while they're being treated. The sensors keep the beam focused on the tumor even while your chest moves from breathing. A somewhat different approach to stereotactic body radiotherapy uses a special frame to hold you very still (what doctors call patient fixation) during the treatment.

SBRT works best on small, well-defined, stage I non–small cell lung cancer tumors. It's most often used as an alternative for patients who aren't good candidates for standard surgery.

Because SBRT equipment is very advanced and expensive, and because radiation oncologists and technologists need special training to use it, the equipment is installed only at major medical centers in the United States. About a hundred medical centers now have the equipment. If your doctor thinks surgery would help you but you're not a good candidate for an operation, ask if stereotactic radiosurgery is a good alternative for you.

Stereotactic Radiosurgery for Brain Metastases

Lung cancer can spread to the brain. Standard external beam radiation treatment can be used to treat these metastases by irradiating the whole brain. There are side effects from whole brain radiation, and the amount of radiation that can be delivered with conventional external beam radiation may not be enough to keep the tumors from coming back. Stereotactic radiosurgery with a gamma knife or linear accelerator (LINAC) can be a good alternative to whole-brain radiation for some brain metastases.

The name *gamma knife* comes from the way this equipment can deliver a very high dose of radiation using gamma rays very precisely to target the tumors and avoid healthy brain tissue. The only difference between gamma knife radiosurgery and LINAC radiosurgery is the design of the equipment. In LINAC radiosurgery, the beam moves constantly around the patient's head; in gamma knife surgery, many beams of radiation from a fixed source converge on the patient's head. If you need stereotactic radiosurgery, the type of equipment that's used makes no difference to the outcome.

Stereotactic radiosurgery for the brain is usually only used for patients who have three or fewer tumors that are fairly small, no larger than three to four centimeters (about one and a half inches).

Only one stereotactic radiosurgery treatment is needed, and there are fewer side effects than from conventional whole-brain radiation. While you're having the treatment, you wear a futuristic-looking special helmet that targets some 200 individual radiation beams at the tumor. A frame holds your head comfortably in place so it can't move. The treatment takes between one and two hours. Patients can generally go home the same day and resume their normal activities quickly.

Stereotactic radiosurgery equipment is very expensive and complex, but today many major medical centers in the United States have it and have staff members who are well trained in using it. If you have brain metastases, ask your doctor if stereotactic radiosurgery is a good alternative to whole brain radiation for you.

Radiofrequency Ablation

Radiofrequency ablation (RFA) is a technique that uses a needle electrode to deliver an electric current to a lung tumor that can't be removed by surgery because the patient isn't a good candidate for an operation. The electrode is put into place through the skin, through a thorascope, or sometimes surgically by opening the chest (thoracostomy). CT scans or other imaging methods are used to guide the electrode to the right place. When the electrode is in position, an electric current is sent through it to create heat that destroys the tumor. Even if RFA can't destroy the tumor completely, it can reduce its size, which may make chemotherapy more effective on the remaining tumor.

RFA isn't as widely used as SBRT because SBRT is less invasive and produces similar results. If you're not a good candidate for lung surgery and want to consider SBRT or RFA as an alternative, talk to your doctor. He or she can help you decide if this is a good idea and can help you find a doctor who can perform one the procedures.

Clinical Trials

How does a new drug become part of standard therapy? Through a long series of clinical trials that test the drug stringently to make sure it is safe, effective, and an improvement over standard treatment. The standard treatments of today, which are the best treatments currently known for cancer, are based on results from past clinical trials.

Clinical trials are research studies that involve people. They're one of the final stages of a very long research process, which may have started years before. The goal of each study is to answer a specific research question about better ways to prevent, diagnose, or treat cancer. In a treatment trial, researchers hope to learn how a new drug or other treatment affects the people who get it.

Clinical trials depend on the volunteer cooperation of patients across the country and sometimes even around the world. For patients, the clinical trial offers high-quality cancer care and the chance to be among the first to benefit if a new treatment is shown to work.

Today there are a number of different types of clinical trials, each with a different set of goals:

- Prevention trials look at new approaches to preventing cancer in the first place and at ways to keep cancer from coming back or new cancers from arising. Prevention trials often involve a vitamin, supplement, or medication doctors think might lower the risk of developing cancer. Most prevention trials involve healthy people who have never had cancer, but some involve cancer patients who want to reduce their risk of recurrence.

- Screening trials test the best way to detect cancer, in the early stages in someone at risk for developing cancer, before it has led to symptoms. Mammography, now standard testing for breast cancer, is an example of a screening test.

- Diagnostic trials explore tests and procedures that may help identify cancer more accurately. Most diagnostic trials involve people who have signs and symptoms of cancer or who have evidence of cancer from imaging.

- Treatment trials are conducted with people who have cancer. The trials test new treatments, such as a new cancer drug, a new combination of drugs, cancer vaccines, a new approach to radiation therapy or surgery, and new treatment methods such as gene therapy.

- Quality of life trials, also know as supportive care trials, look at ways to improve the comfort and quality of life of cancer patients and cancer survivors. These trials study ways to relieve the effects of cancer treatment, such as nausea and sleep disorders.

Some clinical trials include a genetics component, where the researchers look at how an individual's genetic makeup can affect how cancer is detected and diagnosed and responds to treatment. This is a very exciting area of cancer research that we'll discuss more in the next chapter.

For treatment trials, each type of clinical trial has three phases:

1. Phase I trials study how a drug should be given (orally or intravenously, for example), how often is should be taken, and what dose is safe. Usually Phase I trials involve only a small number of patients. In a Phase I cancer study, the patients may not all have the same type of cancer.

2. Phase II trials continue to test the safety of the drug and start to look at how well the new drug works. In most cases, Phase II trials focus on a particular type of cancer and have a larger number of participants.

3. Phase III trials test a new drug, a new drug combination, or a radiation or surgical procedure against the standard treatment. Participants are usually randomly assigned (randomized) to either the standard treatment group or the new treatment group. In either case, you'll be getting the best care for you, because at the very least you'll be getting the current standard of care.

   Phase III trials are usually quite large, often involving hundreds or even thousands of patients with the same type of cancer. These trials generally take place in doctors' offices, clinics, and cancer centers nationwide.

By breaking the testing process down into these slow, careful steps, researchers get reliable information that lets them detect problems very quickly and avoid harming patients. After each phase, the researchers look carefully at the data they have collected and decide whether to move on to the next phase. Often a drug or treatment never gets into Phase III trials because it wasn't shown to be safe or effective. After a Phase III trial, the drug or treatment may turn out to be no better, or even less effective, than standard treatment, but sometimes it turns out to be an improvement, even if the advantage is small. In rare cases, the clinical trial shows such good results that it is ended early so that more patients can receive the treatment. Once the approach taken by the clinical trial has been proven to be safe and effective, it may become part of standard care.

After a treatment has been approved by the FDA and is on the market for all patients, the manufacturer may sponsor a Phase IV trial. The goal of this trial is to look at the side effects, risks, and benefits of the treatment over the long run and in more people than in a Phase III trial.

Is a Clinical Trial Right for You?

Participating in a clinical trial has both benefits and risks. If you're considering being part of a trial, you need to understand both to make the right decision for you. Clinical trials have some significant benefits:

- Access to promising new treatments that usually aren't available except in a clinical trial.
- The new drug or treatment under study may be better than standard treatment—you could be among the first to benefit.

- By participating in the trial, you get regular and careful medical attention from the doctors and other members of the research team.

- Results from this study, even if they're negative, will contribute to future research and help future patients.

Against the upside of a clinical trial is the downside:

- The new drugs or treatments under study aren't always proven to be better than standard treatment.

- Despite careful earlier testing, a new drug or treatment may have unexpected side effects or risks. The side effects and risks may be worse than those of standard care.

- If you are in a randomized trial, you can't choose which approach to receive.

- You may have to see your doctor more often than if you aren't in a clinical trial.

To participate in a clinical trial, you'll need to meet the trial's eligibility criteria—a set of guidelines that describes the characteristics that everyone in the trial has to have. These vary quite a bit from trial to trial. In cancer treatment trials, the criteria usually specify a particular type and stage of cancer and the treatments you've already received. By enrolling only people with similar characteristics, researchers get more meaningful results and minimize the risk that someone will get worse by being in the trial.

Before you enter a clinical trial, you'll be given all the important facts about the trial in writing, including the goal of the study and the possible risks and benefits. This is called informed consent, and it's designed to make sure you know what to expect from your participation. Once you've decided to go ahead, you'll be asked to sign an informed consent form. Signing the form doesn't mean you have to stay in the study. You're free to leave the study at any time for any reason.

If you're considering a clinical trial, you're bound to have a lot of questions. Some important ones to ask include these:

- What is the purpose of this study?
- How long will the study last?
- What are the possible short-term benefits for me?
- What are the possible long-term benefits for me?
- What are the short-term risks, such as unexpected side effects?
- Are there any possible long-term risks, such as delayed side effects?
- What other treatment options are available for me?
- How do the risks and benefits of the study compare to my other options?
- Who will be in charge of my care? Can I still see my regular doctors?
- What follow-up will there be after the study?
- Can I talk to someone already in the study?

If your doctor can't answer all your questions, arrange to talk with a study coordinator, who can give you additional information.

Finding Clinical Trials

Many clinical trials are sponsored by the National Cancer Institute (NCI), which is part of the federal National Institutes of Health (NIH). Other government agencies, such as the U.S. Department of Veterans Affairs, also sponsor clinical trials. So do drug companies, medical institutions, and foundations, such as the American Lung Association, the American Cancer Society, the National Lung Cancer Partnership, and the Lung Cancer Research Foundation.

To find a clinical trial that's right for you, start by asking your doctors. They should have a pretty good idea of the trials that are currently enrolling people like you. In fact, your doctors may suggest a trial even before you ask.

Many trials take place at major cancer centers, and there may not be an appropriate trial near your location. If you meet the criteria for a study, some trials, including many run by the NIH, will provide free treatment, free travel, and help with payment for lodging and other expenses. The study coordinators can help you with payment questions, arrangements, and insurance questions.

A good starting point for finding a trial that's right for you is the National Cancer Institute's website at *www.cancer.gov*. The NIH's website for clinical trials, *www.clinicaltrials.gov*, also lists many opportunities. Many other places also sponsor clinical trials—check the resources section of this book for a list.

Chapter 8

Coming Advances in Lung Cancer Treatment

R esearch into many aspects of lung cancer is very active. In the coming years, we hope to see many advances in screening, imaging, detection, and personalized treatment.

Imaging

Software that will improve our ability to see, identify, measure, and characterize small lung nodules is being developed;

some of these programs are already in clinical trials. Some very exciting developments in this area include the following:

- In dual energy radiography, the computer removes the images of the bony structures from a chest x-ray so that the lung underneath them can be seen more clearly.

- Temporal subtraction radiography lets us compare two chest x-rays taken at different times and highlights changes to make them more obvious to the viewer.

- Computer-aided detection uses software to locate nodules on chest x-rays and CT scans that the viewer might otherwise miss.

- Computer-aided diagnosis uses software to look at features of a lung nodule to predict if it is cancerous or not.

- Volumetric analysis uses programs that measure the size of lung nodules more accurately, telling us not just the diameter of the nodules but also their volume and noting growth rates and changes over time.

The detail now provided by current imaging techniques (e.g., CT scans) is very good, but these scans still have their limits. The detail will continue to improve in coming years and may someday get down to the microscopic level, just as a biopsy now does.

Screening

The results of ongoing large-scale screening trials that use chest imaging to detect lung cancer in people with no symptoms should be available within the next few years. We hope these trials will clarify whether screening for lung cancer using chest imaging works well enough to become part of standard preventative health care. New tests that look for lung cancer markers in the blood and the breath are being developed and may one day be a standard part of screening (see the secton on molecular analysis below).

Bronchoscopy

New technologies for bronchoscopy will become available in the near future:

- Today a bronchoscope is about the thickness of a pencil and can't enter airways that are any narrower than that. Ultrathin bronchoscopes that can reach deeper into the small airways are in development.

- Real-time imaging will guide the bronchoscope and tell us which airways to enter as we do the procedure.

- Narrow-band imaging will show us the changes in blood vessels in the airways that may signal the start of cancer.

- Optical coherence tomography will allow us to see structures down to the microscopic level during bronchoscopy.

The more we can see deeper into the lung using the bronchoscope, the more we can do to detect lung cancer early, get good biopsy samples for diagnosis and staging, and possibly treat cancer in its earliest stages.

Molecular Analysis

The more we can learn about the molecular basis of cancer—what happens inside a cell to make it cancerous—the more we can advance the areas of lung cancer prevention, detection, and treatment. Molecular analysis of tumor tissue, blood, and breath will lead to the discovery of biomarkers for lung cancer. Biomarkers can be developed into tests that will help us predict who will develop lung cancer; which cancers are likely to be aggressive and, therefore, more likely to benefit from aggressive approaches to therapy; and which medications an individual person's cancer is likely to respond to. They may even lead to the discovery of new cancer pathways and targeted therapies.

Advances in molecular analysis and biomarker development have been coming fast in recent years. Areas that are being looked at include study of the gene profile of tumor tissue and blood, the protein patterns in tumor tissue and blood, the detection of antibodies to tumor-associated antigens (proteins) in the blood, the detection of tumor cells circulating in the blood, the patterns of an internal cellular material (called microRNA) in the blood, the detection of alterations in the DNA floating in the blood (one example is called DNA methylation) that affect its function, the patterns of volatile organic compounds in the breath, and the composition of exhaled breath condensate. One or many of these basic scientific advances is certain to find a place in clinical lung cancer management in the near future.

Personalized Treatment

Every patient with lung cancer is different, and today doctors do all they can to tailor treatment to the individual, taking into account your type of cancer, the stage, and your overall health. In the near future, your treatment will probably be individualized to a much greater degree using advances in molecular analysis and biomarker development. By looking at the genetic and other characteristics of your cancer at the cellular level, your doctor will know if you're likely to respond well to standard chemotherapy and, if so, to which combination of drugs, and whether you're a good candidate for targeted therapies that block a process within the cancer cell. Doctors will be able to predict which drugs will work best for you and combine them in ways tailored just for you. This will help eliminate some of the educated guesswork that is almost inevitable with cancer treatment.

It's also possible that in the future, researchers will be able to look at cells from your lung and detect the earliest molecular changes that mean cancer is getting started. Molecular analysis is one possible future way to screen for early lung cancer. Looking at the molecular characteristics of your cancer cells may also help predict the course of your disease and point more accurately toward the treatment that will be best for you.

Treatment

In the very near future, we hope that personalized treatment based on molecular analysis and targeted medications will become standard. New medications and new combinations of available treatments will be tested. We'll have new, even more high-tech ways to deliver optimal radiation therapy. Improvements in treatment to minimize side effects and palliate the symptoms of advanced disease will continue to come quickly.

Agents currently in study for the treatment of lung cancer include additional receptor tyrosine kinases (such as the EGFR inhibitors), nonreceptor tyrosine kinases, other angiogenesis inhibitors, proteosome inhibitors, therapies directed at tumor-associated antigens (such as vaccines and means to deliver radioisotopes to tumors), therapies targeting cell survival pathways and retinoid signaling pathways, and means to sensitize the tumor to the effects of chemotherapies.

Hope for the Future

The very promising developments in the evaluation and management of lung cancer are a reason for great hope for lung cancer patients. Lung cancer patients today have good reason to feel more hopeful than ever.

Chapter 9

Maintaining Quality of Life

Today we can do so much more to help lung cancer patients than even a few years ago—and in the future, we will be able to do even more. But for all the promise of the progress that is happening, advanced lung cancer remains difficult to cure. Additional therapy after your initial treatment can do a great deal to improve your quality of life and prolong survival. And when active treatment is no longer helpful or desired, today we have many ways to provide comfort care for this last period of life. Most people with terminal lung cancer can remain at home with their loved ones as pain-free, dignified, and comfortable as possible.

Comfort Care

Palliative care, also known as comfort care or supportive care, is treatment that is meant to help maintain a good quality of life for lung cancer patients whose disease can't be cured, only managed. From the day a cancer patient is diagnosed, quality of life is an integral part of cancer care. No cancer patient should have untreated pain, discomfort, or distress.

The goal of palliative care is to provide patient-centered care that prevents and relieves suffering and supports the best possible quality of life for patients and their loved ones. Palliative care focuses not just on treating pain and other distressing symptoms—it also offers spiritual and emotional support that is sensitive to the patient's beliefs and culture.

Pain Management

Advanced cancer patients often experience pain, sometimes severe, from the tumor itself, metastases (especially those that go to bones), complications of the tumor, or treatment. Fortunately, today's treatment arsenal gives us many very effective ways to relieve cancer pain.

Radiation Therapy and Chemotherapy

Radiation treatment is a mainstay of palliative treatment for advanced lung cancer. If the cancer has spread to the bones or the brain, for example, radiation therapy can help relieve symptoms such as pain and nausea.

Palliative radiation is given as needed to relieve the problem. The area that gets the radiation, the dose, and how many treatments are needed depend of the location of the pain, the size of the tumor, and how much radiation the patient has already received from earlier treatments. Often several treatments are given over several days; most patients won't need to do daily treatments for several weeks on end, as they would with external beam radiation therapy at an earlier stage of the disease.

Chemotherapy can be used to help shrink tumors that are causing pain by pressing on other parts of the body or shortness of breath from blocking an airway. Palliative chemotherapy isn't meant to cure the cancer, only to relieve symptoms. For patients who receive chemotherapy, the toxic side effects of the chemotherapy and their impact on the quality of life need to be weighed against the potential response and resultant relief of pain and other symptoms. Sometimes relief can come from other methods, such as pain medication. Chemotherapy near the end of life is a very difficult decision—there are no easy answers.

Pain Medication

We've discussed pain management with medication while you're in treatment in detail in chapter 6. The same concepts apply to comfort care. The crucial point to remember is that cancer pain can almost always be relieved. There's no reason for any cancer patient to have untreated or undertreated pain.

The pain from advanced cancer, especially if it has spread to the bones, usually needs strong drugs for relief. Opioids, also called narcotics, are generally prescribed for moderate to severe pain. Commonly prescribed opioids include the following:

- Codeine
- Fentanyl (Actiq, Duragesic, Fentora, Sublimaze)
- Hydromorphone (Dilaudid)
- Levorphanol (Levo-Dromoran)
- Meperidine (Demerol)
- Methadone (Symoron, Amidol)
- Morphine
- Oxycodone (OxyContin)
- Oxymorphone (Opana)

Side effects of opioids include constipation, drowsiness, nausea, and vomiting. Most patients get over the side effects within a few days. If the side effects continue, tell your doctor. Often changing the dose, switching to a different drug, or adding an additional drug to control the side effects helps the problem.

Over time, your opioid dose may need to be increased or changed to give you the same relief. This may be caused by worsening pain from the cancer. Another common reason is that you have built up a tolerance to the drug and need a larger dose or need to take it more often. You might also need a stronger drug at this point. If your opioid medication isn't working well for you any more, talk to your doctor about what to do. Don't increase the dose of the drug or how often you take it on your own.

Constipation from opioids is a very common side effect that can easily be managed. Don't be embarrassed to discuss this with your doctor—almost every patient who takes these drugs will have the same problem. In fact, your doctor may prescribe a mild laxative and stool softeners when you start taking the drugs to help keep the problem from happening. Drinking more fluids and eating foods high in fiber help; fiber supplements such as psyllium (Metamucil), taken with plenty of water, are often very helpful. Getting as much exercise as you can also helps.

Drowsiness from opioids can be a problem, though it often goes away after a few days. If you feel drowsy from the drug or for any other reason, be very careful to avoid falls. Don't go up and down stairs by yourself, for example, and be cautious getting in and out of bed and up and down from chairs. Don't do anything where you need to be alert, like driving. If your drowsiness doesn't go away within a week or so, call your doctor. You may need a smaller dose or a different drug.

Nausea and vomiting from opioids also usually go away after a few days. The nausea is often described as being like seasickness, and moving around can make it worse. Try staying in bed or sitting quietly for an hour or so after taking your pain medication. If the symptoms don't go away within a few days, call your doctor. You may need to take an antinausea drug or switch to a different painkiller.

Your pain medicine will work best if you take it as directed. Take the medicine on a regular schedule, even if your pain isn't that bad. The drug may not work as well if you wait until the pain returns to take it. Unless your doctor tells you to, don't split, chew, or crush the pills. Often, to help patients save money on drug costs, doctors will prescribe a larger dose of a medicine so that you can split the pills to get the lower dose that's right for you. Unless that's the case, though, don't split the pills—you could end up taking too little to help. If you crush or chew the pills, your body will absorb the drug quickly, and you could end up getting too much of it too fast. If you are crushing the pills because you have trouble swallowing them, let your doctor know. Many drugs can be given as a liquid, in a form that dissolves quickly in your mouth, as a suppository, or as a patch you wear on your skin.

Other Treatments for Pain

Drugs such as corticosteroids can often be helpful for pain caused by swelling. Drugs that affect bone turnover are sometimes tried for helping bone pain from metastases. These drugs have side effects that can include bone, joint, and muscle pain. Talk to your doctor about the pros and cons of using them.

Interventions are sometimes recommended to treat severe pain that isn't being helped much by drugs. If that's the case, your doctor may refer you to a specialist in pain management. One safe method that can be used to relieve pain is a nerve block. This controls pain by injecting a local anesthetic, such as lidocaine, into or around the nerves that carry pain or into the spinal column. Sometimes a drug that destroys the nerve is injected (neurolysis) so the nerve can't transmit the pain signal any longer.

Complications of Advanced Lung Cancer

Someone with advanced lung cancer may develop some serious complications that cause discomfort and distress.

Fortunately, we can usually treat these complications easily and keep the patient functioning well.

If you develop any of the problems discussed below, call your doctor. Some problems, such as a blood clot in the lung, are oncologic emergencies that need immediate attention. Any sudden or unexpected symptom is cause for concern. Call your doctor at once or go to the emergency room

Shortness of Breath and Difficulty Breathing

A very common problem for people with advanced lung cancer is shortness of breath or difficult, painful breathing (dyspnea). Difficulty breathing can have many causes, so it's important to discuss the problem with your doctor. In general, treatment with drugs or other methods is based on the underlying cause of the breathing problem.

Blocked Airways. Sometimes patients with advanced lung cancer have shortness of breath and pain because the tumor is narrowing or blocking an airway. Depending on the type of cancer, how large the tumor is, and where it is located, your doctor may suggest one of several different treatment options.

People with small cell lung cancer can have narrowed airways because the tumor has infiltrated the lining of the breathing tubes. SCLC is very responsive to both chemotherapy and radiation therapy, so treatment usually helps with breathing problems.

Blocked airways from the tumor growing inside the tubes can be a problem for people with any type of lung cancer, particularly squamous cell carcinoma. External beam radiation to the chest is an effective treatment that helps to open up the airway so that the patient can breathe better. Chemotherapy can also help, but the response is slower. If external beam radiation hasn't helped or isn't possible, brachytherapy (also called internal radiation or endobronchial radiotherapy), can be used. Brachytherapy may be done in a radiation oncologist's office or in the hospital. A bronchoscope is used to insert a thin tube called a catheter into the affected area. Radioactive material is then sent into the catheter and placed next to the tumor. The radioactive material delivers radiation just to the area nearby. The radiation kills the cancer cells and opens the airway. You're not radioactive from the treatment, so you can resume your normal activities right away.

If radiation therapy doesn't help, can't be done, or is going to take too long to have an effect, treatment through a bronchoscope (camera inserted into the airways) may be offered. One bronchoscopic approach is to open up the tube by inserting a stent—an expandable tube that props the airway open. In most cases, a wire mesh tube that expands outward once it's inserted into the airway is used. The stent is put into place using a bronchoscope while you are under general anesthesia. Afterward, most patients recover quickly and can't feel the stent. It can stay in place permanently.

Other bronchoscopic approaches for a blocked airway include laser therapy, where a laser beam is used to burn away the tumor, or electrocautery, which uses an electric current to destroy the tumor in the blocked area. These are often used in combination with stent placement. During these treatments, you're sedated or have general anesthesia. You can often go home the same day or after just an overnight stay in the hospital.

Often shortness of breath is because the patient's overall lung function is poor due to other health problems, such as emphysema, in addition to the lung cancer. Medications to treat the underlying lung problem can be helpful. Other causes of shortness of breath include pleural effusions and blood clots (we'll talk about those later on in this chapter).

Supplemental Oxygen. Sometimes a patient's lungs aren't working well enough to keep up a normal level of oxygen in the blood. When your blood oxygen level drops too low (below 88 percent saturation), your doctor may prescribe wearable oxygen for you, which may help you breathe more easily.

Supplemental oxygen, delivered through a nasal cannula, can do a great deal to help the patient breathe more easily and relax. The nasal cannula is a lightweight, two-pronged device that fits into the nostrils and is connected to the thin plastic tubing that carries the oxygen. The tubing is flexible and lightweight. To stay in place, it usually rests on the ears. The nasal cannula is very comfortable and unobtrusive—patients can talk, eat, drink, move around, and sleep comfortably while wearing it.

It's easy to use supplemental oxygen at home. The oxygen may be provided as compressed or liquid gas in a large, heavy cylinder, but in most cases, an oxygen concentrator is used. The oxygen concentrator is a compact, very quiet machine that runs on household electricity. It pulls oxygen from the air, concentrates it, and stores it until you need to breathe it. Extra tubing can be attached so you can move around easily— you can even be in a different room. Oxygen concentrators are very convenient because they don't have to be refilled.

Oxygen concentrators run on electricity, so you need to have an oxygen cylinder as backup in case of a power failure.

For traveling outside the home, a small, portable oxygen cylinder can be carried with you.

If you need supplemental oxygen at home, your doctor will prescribe it and help you arrange for it. The equipment is usually provided and maintained by a medical equipment company; the cost is usually covered by health insurance.

Coughing. Chronic coughing from lung cancer can be uncomfortable. It can keep you from sleeping, and it can make dyspnea worse. The treatment for coughing depends on the underlying cause. It could be from a common cause of coughing, such as postnasal drip; from chronic obstructive pulmonary disease, such as emphysema; from airway involvement with the tumor; or from the effects of radiation therapy (pneumonitis). Treatment of the cause of the cough is the most helpful intervention. When the cause can't be eliminated, then cough suppressants can be helpful.

Your doctor may prescribe a cough-suppressing medicine containing codeine, hydrocodone, or dextromethorphan. Drugs that help break up mucus and help you cough it up, such as guaifenesin, may also be used.

Coughing up a lot of blood (hemoptysis), especially if it happens suddenly, needs immediate treatment. In advanced cancer, the bleeding is usually caused because small blood vessels around the tumor have ruptured or because the tumor has invaded a blood vessel in the lung. Severe, sudden bleeding can occur if the tumor breaks into a large blood vessel. Radiation treatment can sometimes help stop the bleeding. Another approach is to block the bleeding vessels by inserting a tiny metal coil or type of foam into the bleeding blood vessels using a thin catheter snaked into them (called angiography with embolization).

Malignant Pleural or Pericardial Effusion. A buildup of fluid in the pleural cavity (the space in the chest surrounding each lung) because the cancer has spread to that area is called a malignant pleural effusion. It can cause shortness of breath, dry cough, chest pain, and a feeling of heaviness in the chest. To help you feel better, your doctor will probably drain off the fluid. One way to do this is called a thoracentesis—inserting a small needle between the ribs into the pleural cavity to remove the fluid. Another method of fluid removal is called tube thoracostomy. The doctor inserts a small tube into the fluid-filled area to drain it.

Draining off the fluid often only helps for a short time, until the fluid collects again. To help keep this from happening, your doctor may perform a pleurodesis through the tube to close off the pleural sac so fluid can't build up inside it: after the fluid is removed, a substance that makes the sac close is inserted into the space through the chest tube. Alternatively, the doctor may look into the space around the lungs using a small camera before removing the fluid and doing the pleurodesis. In some cases, the doctor may choose to leave a small tube in place so that the fluid can be drained every few days or as needed.

When fluid from the cancer builds up in the sac around the heart, it's called a malignant pericardial effusion. The excess fluid pressing on your heart can cause shortness of breath, coughing, chest pain, swelling in the upper abdomen, difficulty breathing while lying flat, and extreme tiredness. Another symptom is hiccups that won't go away.

To relieve the symptoms, your doctor will probably try to drain off the fluid by inserting a needle into the sac, a procedure called a pericardiocentesis. Sometimes a surgical incision is made through the chest into the pericardium to insert a drainage tube. It's also possible to use other, more invasive procedures to help. Many patients with a malignant pericardial effusion, however, are near the end of life and may not want or be strong enough for these procedures.

Blood Clots

Deep Vein Thrombosis. People with lung cancer are at high risk of deep vein thrombosis (DVT)—a dangerous blood clot that forms inside a vein deep in the legs. Sometimes the clot can travel to the lungs, where it can cause serious symptoms and even death.

Aside from the cancer itself, risks for developing deep vein thrombosis include cigarette smoking, recent surgery, sitting for a long time (as in a long plane ride), and prolonged bed rest. Some targeted therapy drugs, such as bevacizumab (Avastin), may also increase your risk of blood clots.

The most common symptom of a deep vein clot in the leg is swelling in the affected leg. The leg may also turn red and feel warmer than the other leg, and there may be some pain. Call your doctor at once if you notice any symptoms of DVT. A painless ultrasound examination of the leg usually reveals where the clot is.

Treatment for DVT usually involves blood thinners, such as warfarin (Coumadin) or heparin. Treatment helps prevent bigger clots from developing and travelling to the lungs. These drugs need to be used very cautiously, especially in patients with advanced cancer, because they increase your overall risk of bleeding.

Preventing DVT whenever possible is very important for lung cancer patients. One important measure is to move the legs by walking, gentle stretching, and simple exercises that can be done even while lying in bed. If you're in the hospital and don't feel up to being active, you may be given low doses of a blood thinner by injection to prevent clots.

Pulmonary Embolus. A blood clot that travels to the lung is called a pulmonary embolus. The clot usually blocks an artery in the lung. The most common symptom is sudden shortness of breath. You may also have chest pain. The pain can be very sharp or stabbing, or feel like an ache on one side of your chest. It may get worse when you take a deep breath or cough. Other symptoms include a sudden cough, rapid breathing, and rapid heart rate. You may also experience the symptoms of a deep vein thrombosis, such as a leg that's swollen, as described above.

Blood clots are very serious for anyone but especially for lung cancer patients. *If you have symptoms of a pulmonary embolus, don't delay—go to the emergency room at once.* Prompt treatment can help prevent death from the clot.

Treatment for a pulmonary embolus is usually with blood thinners such as warfarin or heparin. You may need to continue to take these drugs indefinitely.

Superior Vena Cava Syndrome

Tumors in the chest can sometimes press on a large vein called the superior vena cava, which carries blood back to the heart. If the vein is blocked, the patient develops superior vena cava syndrome (SVCS). The symptoms of SVCS usually develop slowly and include difficulty breathing and coughing. The face, neck, upper body, and arms may gradually swell up.

Mild superior vena cava syndrome may not need a lot of treatment. Keeping the upper body raised higher than the lower body helps with coughing and difficulty breathing. For more severe cases, shrinking the tumor where it presses on the vein can help. Radiation therapy and chemotherapy may be used, depending on the individual and what treatment he or she is already getting. Inserting a stent into the blocked area of the vein to prop it open helps some patients.

Spinal Cord Compression

Lung cancer that has metastasized to the spinal column (backbone) can sometimes grow large enough to press on the spinal nerves. When the nerves are compressed by a tumor pressing on them, severe back pain and weakness and loss of sensation in the legs result. Spinal cord compression needs immediate treatment to relieve the pain and prevent permanent damage to the nerves that control the lower part of the body. Call your doctor at once or go to the emergency room if you have symptoms of spinal compression. Radiation therapy and medications can usually relieve the problem.

Hypercalcemia

Hypercalcemia, or too much calcium in the blood, is sometimes a problem for people with lung cancer, particularly if they have a paraneoplastic syndrome from squamous type non–small cell lung cancer (see chapter 2) or if they have many metastases to the bones from advanced cancer. For complex reasons, the body absorbs too much calcium from the bones, and the kidneys can't excrete it.

Symptoms of hypercalcemia include feeling very tired, having trouble thinking clearly, lack of appetite, frequent urination, increased thirst, constipation, and nausea and vomiting. Because these symptoms resemble symptoms from other causes, such as pain drugs, hypercalcemia may not be noticed at first. Many people with advanced cancer have hypercalcemia but don't know it because their symptoms are very mild and don't really need to be treated. It's only when more serious symptoms appear, such as extreme tiredness or lassitude, that treatment may be needed.

Treating mild hypercalcemia usually involves giving the patient IV fluids, because dehydration often contributes to the problem. For moderate to severe hypercalcemia, IV fluids also help. Drugs that slow the turnover of bone, such as the biphosphonates, are sometimes used to help. Some patients who are near the end of life and have hypercalcemia will choose not to treat it. Untreated severe hypercalcemia leads to loss of consciousness, coma, and death, usually within a few days.

Staying well hydrated, by drinking enough fluids and controlling vomiting, helps prevent hypercalcemia.

Mental Confusion and Delirium

Patients with advanced lung cancer may experience periods of mental confusion and delirium that cause changes in normal behavior. The mental confusion and delirium affect the patient's ability to think, pay attention, be aware of his or her surroundings, and remember things. The patient may also

Oncologic Emergencies

Some complications from advanced lung cancer can be serious and need immediate treatment. Call your doctor or go to the emergency room for any of these problems:

- Symptoms of severe hypercalcemia
- Severe back pain or weakness or loss of sensation in the legs
- Coughing up a lot of blood
- Seizure
- Difficulty being awoken or loss of consciousness
- Depressed breathing with very low blood pressure
- Swelling, redness, or warmth in just one leg
- Sudden or unusual shortness of breath
- Sudden, severe chest pain under the breastbone or on one side

seem disoriented, experience emotional or mood swings, and have an altered pattern of sleeping and waking. Patients with delirium may also go in and out of consciousness.

Sometimes people with mental confusion or delirium can become very agitated or even violent. These symptoms can be very distressing for the family and caregivers. They may also be dangerous to the patient, who may fall or try to do things, such as climb out of bed, that can cause harm.

Delirium and mental confusion usually have underlying causes that can be treated. Metastases to the brain are a potential cause of the symptoms. Treating the metastases if possible, as discussed in earlier chapters, may help. Some

Talking about Your Final Wishes

Talking about death is very difficult, yet talking about it can also help someone with advanced cancer feel better emotionally. Making sure your loved ones know your final wishes, also called advance directives, can lead to greater peace of mind. A living will spells out your wishes regarding your medical care, including whether you want to refuse life-prolonging treatment if death is near. Another important advance directive is a health care power of attorney. In this document, you name someone you trust to act for you and make decisions about your medical care if you are unable to do so. A health care power of attorney does not have to be a family member.

Advance directives can be withdrawn or changed by the patient at any time. The laws about advance directives and their wording vary from state to state, but in general you don't need a lawyer to prepare these documents. Free standardized forms for a living will and health care power of attorney are easily available—check your state's Department of Health or Department of Aging, ask at the hospital, or check the resources section at the back of this book.

Many patients also write a letter of intent that clarifies their wishes about whom they want to care for them in their final days, what kind of funeral service they want, who will take care of their pets, and other details that are important to them.

medications cause delirium; stopping or reducing the dose of the medication may be necessary. Other treatable causes of delirium include dehydration, an infection, hypercalcemia, and hyponatremia (too little sodium in the blood). Very near the end of life, delirium is fairly common and can't be treated. Sedation to help relieve the agitation may be considered. This is a difficult decision that needs to be taken in consultation with the family and the care team.

Complementary and Alternative Therapies

Many lung cancer patients consider complementary and alternative therapies (CAM) as part of their treatment. Some of these can be helpful, but all complementary and alternative therapies must always be used very cautiously and always in consultation with your doctor.

Complementary therapies are generally those that are used alongside your regular medical care. Alternative therapies are generally those that are used instead of regular medical care.

Complementary treatments aren't curative. Instead, they're nondrug methods that are used to help you feel better. Ginger or peppermint tea, for instance, can help relieve nausea. Meditation and guided imagery can help reduce stress and help you sleep better, and acupuncture can help some people get pain relief. Before using any complementary method, discuss it with your doctor first. While some therapies, such as acupuncture, are usually safe and may even be covered by your health insurance, many other complementary therapies have never been tested, and it's not known if they really help—some could even be harmful. Many herbal remedies, including those from traditional Chinese and Ayurvedic medicine, need to be used very, very cautiously.

Alternative treatments are often touted as cancer "cures" instead of standard medical care. Unlike standard medical care, these treatments haven't been proven safe and effective in clinical trials. They may have dangerous and even life-threatening side effects. Even worse, if you follow these treatments instead of receiving standard medical care, you may lose precious time. While you're following alternative treatments that are very unlikely to help, your cancer is growing, making it less likely that medical treatment will help.

The promoters of alternative cancer treatments often count on your natural desire to do all you can to fight your cancer—and on your very natural desire to avoid the unpleasant side effects of standard medical treatment. If treatments such as chemotherapy aren't working for you any more, you may be willing to try anything that claims to help.

While many of the people promoting alternative cancer treatments are sincere,, others aren't. They're willing to take advantage of your health situation to charge you large amounts of money for treatments that don't work and may well be harmful.

Always discuss frankly any alternative treatment you might be considering with your doctor. To avoid fraudulent cancer treatments, look for these red flags:

- Does the treatment promise to "cure" all cancer?

- Are you told that the treatment won't work unless you stop all standard medical treatment?

- Does the treatment involve ingredients or practices that only a few sources, individuals, or clinics can provide?

- Does the advertising use words like *miracle cure, natural,* or *secret?*

- Does the advertising present a lot of testimonials from patients but not much scientific evidence?

- Do you have to travel to another country to get the treatment?

Any of these red flags is a sign that a fraudster is at work. Protect your health and your wallet and stay away from alternative treatments for cancer.

Hospice Care

As lung cancer progresses and a patient no longer has effective options for fighting the tumor, treatment often shifts from prolonging life to maintaining the best possible quality of life. This means continuing palliative care to control pain and other symptoms and taking steps to keep the patient as comfortable as possible. By definition, palliative care seeks to ease symptoms without curing the underlying disease.

When patients have only months or weeks to live, hospice care can be very valuable for helping them receive the best supportive care and live out the rest of their lives with dignity. The concept behind hospice care is to offer comprehensive palliative care for people who are terminally ill; most patients are no longer receiving treatment that is meant to be curative. The hospice care team works closely with the patient's own doctors and family to coordinate care.

The hospice team of trained professionals offers pain management, expert care for other symptoms, and emotional and spiritual support for both the patient and the family. The services available through hospice programs generally include doctor services, pain management, regular home visits from registered nurses and licensed practical nurses, medical equipment such as hospital beds and oxygen equipment, and help from specialists such as physical therapists. Hospice volunteers are often available to give family members some time away from the patient to take care of their own needs. Although residential hospices are available, one of the great advantages of hospice is that it comes to you. Patients can remain in the familiar surroundings of their own homes with their families and loved ones. In almost all cases, health insurance covers the costs of hospice. To find a hospice program in your community, check the resources section of this book.

Hope, Now and in the Future

Today we can do a great deal to help patients live well with lung cancer. New treatments help patients live longer and better, with fewer side effects and little pain. The latest developments in diagnosis and treatment all give hope for curing the cancer, or prolonging survival and maintaining a good quality of life even as the end of life approaches. Going forward, we hope new methods will help us to prevent lung cancer from developing or let us detect lung cancer early, when it is most treatable. We also look ahead to a time when every patient with lung cancer will receive personalized treatment based on his or her genetic profile, treatments will be increasingly effective and have fewer side effects. Our ever-improving understanding of how cancer develops and grows means that the future for lung cancer management is brighter than ever.

Acknowledgments

I would like to thank the Cleveland Clinic, Chairman of the Respiratory Institute Dr. Herbert Wiedemann, and Kaplan Publishing for the opportunity to write this book. My sincere gratitude is extended to Sheila Buff for working with me to create this book and to Shannon Berning for her support. I appreciate the education I have received from my local and distant lung cancer colleagues. Finally, I want to recognize the sacrifices my wife and daughter have made to allow me to work on this book.

Appendix A

Quit Smoking Now!

On April 5, 2005, beloved network news anchor Peter Jennings announced on the air that he had been diagnosed with lung cancer. Jennings had smoked for decades, quit for 20 years, and started smoking again in the aftermath of the September 11, 2001, attacks. He died four months later. He was 67.

Some smokers have pointed to Jennings's death as a reason to continue smoking. After all, they say, he quit and still died of lung cancer. They couldn't be more wrong. By quitting for 20 years, Jennings probably delayed his lung cancer. Starting to smoke again could have accelerated the disease.

Stopping smoking at any age, no matter how long you've smoked, helps your overall health and reduces your risk of lung cancer. If you've smoked for a long time and quit, however, your risk of getting lung cancer won't ever drop to that of someone who never smoked. It will still drop, however—ten years after quitting, your risk of lung cancer will be one-third to one-half lower than the risk to people who continue to smoke.

The Risks of Secondhand Smoke

Studies have shown that nonsmoker spouses of smokers have a 24 to 30 percent greater risk of developing lung cancer than do spouses of nonsmokers. Secondhand smokers are exposed to the same cancer-causing agents as smokers, although in weaker amounts.

Inhaling tobacco smoke from other smokers sharing living or working areas (also called passive smoking or environmental tobacco smoking) increases the risk of getting lung cancer by at least 20 percent and causes an estimated 3,000 lung cancer deaths annually. The risks of secondhand smoke are why smoking is now banned in just about every public place, including restaurants, bars, and hospitals. Secondhand smoke is dangerous at home, too. Children living with smokers are at greater risk for asthma, ear infections, and respiratory problems.

Dangers of Cigars, Smokeless Tobacco, and Marijuana

Cigar smoke contains the same toxic compounds as cigarette smoke, making cigars just as dangerous. Some premium cigars contain the tobacco equivalent of an entire pack of cigarettes. Not only are cigar smokers at risk of lung cancer, they also are at high risk for cancers of the oral cavity, including the lips, gums, tongue, mouth, and throat.

Chewing tobacco and snuff are often called smokeless tobacco. Because they don't create smoke that's inhaled, they're not associated with lung cancer—but smokeless tobacco is far more dangerous when it comes to other cancers, especially cancers of the oral cavity.

What about smoking marijuana? The risk here is a little less clear—one major study from 2006 showed no increased risk of lung cancer among regular and even heavy marijuana smokers. But in 2008, another, more carefully controlled study suggested that smoking just one marijuana joint a day is the equivalent of smoking a pack of cigarettes a day, with the same increased risk of lung cancer.

New Antismoking Legislation

In 2009, new federal antismoking legislation gave the Food and Drug Administration (FDA) increased power to regulate the content, marketing, and advertising of cigarettes and other tobacco products. The agency will be able to limit the amount of nicotine in tobacco products, but it won't be able to ban nicotine or cigarettes. The new law allows the FDA to prohibit tobacco companies from marketing their products to teenagers and calls for much tougher warning labels on tobacco packages. The law also prohibits the use of terms such as *light* or *mild,* which suggest that these products have a smaller health risk.

Quit and Quit Now

Most health problems related to cigarette smoking, including lung cancer, can be reduced by stopping smoking. In fact, smokers who quit reduce their risk of lung cancer death by 30 to 50 percent after ten years. Smokers who quit before age 50 have half the risk of dying in the next 16 years compared with people who continue to smoke. And women who stop smoking before becoming pregnant or who quit in the first three months of pregnancy can reverse the risk of low birth weight for the baby and reduce other pregnancy-associated risks. Quitting smoking also greatly reduces the risk of developing other smoking-related diseases, such as cancers of the oral cavity, esophageal cancer, heart disease, stroke, emphysema, and chronic bronchitis.

But as so many current and past smokers can attest, quitting isn't easy. There's no one way to quit that works for everyone, but here are some helpful tips from the experts at the Cleveland Clinic:

- Begin a smoking cessation program through a health care provider in your community. The program should help you pick a date to stop smoking and prepare for it and help you know what triggers your urge to smoke. Many local hospitals and other organizations, such as local chapters of the American Lung Association, offer free smoking cessation programs.

- Make a list of your reasons for quitting and read it frequently.

- Don't focus on what's missing. Think about what will be gained—better health.

- Consider using a nicotine replacement product, such as nicotine patches or gum, to help you quit. Ask your doctor about a nicotine-free prescription medication, such as Zyban (bupropion) or Chantix (varenicline), that can help.

- Try to break the connection between smoking and certain activities, such as having a cigarette on your coffee break.

- When the urge to smoke occurs, take a deep breath, hold it for ten seconds, then release it slowly. Just a brief pause can help the urge pass quickly.

- When the urge for a cigarette strikes, eat something instead—preferably a low-calorie, healthful food. Pop a small piece of sugar-free hard candy, chew sugar-free gum, or have something nonalcoholic and sugar-free to drink, such as a diet soda.

- Keep your hands busy with something other than a cigarette. Doodle, knit, play a video game, work on a hobby.

- Don't carry cigarettes, a lighter, or matches.

- Drink plenty of fluids. If you usually smoke a cigarette with alcohol or coffee, though, cut back on these drinks—they'll trigger your desire to smoke.

- Exercise more—it's good for you, and it helps you relax.

- Get support for quitting by telling others about your milestones.

It's not easy to quit smoking, but very few things that you do in life will be more important to your health. There's a chance that your first try won't be successful—many smokers need two or three tries before they can quit completely. But remember, it's also never too late to quit. Keep trying.

What Happens When You Quit Smoking?

After 20 minutes:
- Your blood pressure and pulse decrease.

After 8 hours:
- The carbon monoxide level in your blood returns to normal.
- Oxygen levels in your blood increase.

After 24 hours:
- Your chance of a heart attack decreases.

After 48 hours:
- Your nerve endings adjust to the absence of nicotine.
- Your ability to taste and smell begin to return.

After 72 hours:
- Your bronchial tubes relax.

After 2 weeks to 3 months:
- Your circulation improves.
- Your exercise tolerance improves.

After 1 to 9 months:
- Coughing, sinus congestion, fatigue, and shortness of breath decrease.
- Your overall energy level increases.

After 1 year:
- Your risk of heart disease decreases to half that of a current smoker.

(continued)

After 5 years:
- Your risk of stroke is reduced to that of people who have never smoked.

After 10 years:
- Your risk of dying from lung cancer drops to almost the same rate as that of a lifelong nonsmoker.
- Your risk of other cancers—of the mouth, larynx, esophagus, bladder, kidney, and pancreas—decreases.

Appendix B

Resources for More Information

General Information about Lung Cancer

An excellent starting point for more information about lung cancer is

National Cancer Institute (NCI)
800-4-CANCER (800-422-6237)
www.cancer.gov

The NCI offers specific information about lung cancer, as well as valuable information about all aspects of cancer treatment and cancer care. In addition, the comprehensive Physician Data Query (PDQ) base is an excellent source for summaries of the latest published information on cancer detection, treatment, and supportive care. The patient versions of PDQ summaries are written in nontechnical language.

Other good sources of information for people with lung cancer include the following:

American Cancer Society (ACS)
800-ACS-2345 (800-227-2345)
www.cancer.org

Cancer.net (oncologist-approved cancer information
from the American Society of Clinical Oncology)
888-651-3038
www.cancer.net

**Cleveland Clinic Center for Consumer Health
Information**
866-594-2091
http://my.clevelandclinic.org/health

Cleveland Clinic Cancer Answer Line
866-223-8100

LungCancer.org
800-813-4673
www.lungcancer.org

National Comprehensive Cancer Network (NCCN)
888-909-NCCN (888-909-6226)
www.nccn.com

Advanced Directives

State-specific advance directives (living will and health care
power of attorney) can be downloaded from

Caring Connections
800-658-8898
www.caringinfo.org

Clinical Trials

Clinical trials are very important for advancing cancer treatment and may be of benefit to people with lung cancer. Many organizations run clinical trials, and finding one that's appropriate can be challenging. Following are the best starting points for finding an appropriate clinical trial:

CenterWatch
www.centerwatch.com

ClinicalTrials.gov (A service of the U.S. National Institutes of Health)
www.clinicaltrials.gov

Coalition of Cancer Cooperative Groups
877-520-4457
www.cancertrialshelp.org

EmergingMed
877-601-8601
www.emergingmed.com

National Cancer Institute (NCI)
800-4-CANCER (800-422-6237)
www.cancer.gov

Cognitive Behavioral Therapy

Cognitive behavioral therapy can very helpful for both patients and caregivers coping with anxiety, depression, grief, and bereavement. To find a qualified CBT therapist near you, contact

Association for Behavioral and Cognitive Therapies
(212) 647-1890
www.abct.org

Complementary and Alternative Treatment (CAM)

The National Center for Complementary and Alternative Medicine is a part of the National Institutes of Health. It's a very good starting point for accurate, scientific information about CAM:

National Center for Complementary and Alternative
    Medicine (NCCAM)
888-644-6226
www.nccam.nih.gov

Financial Assistance

Cancer treatment can be very expensive. Your doctors and hospital will do all they can to help you with financial assistance. These organizations may also be able to help:

NeedyMeds
www.needymeds.org

Patient Advocate Foundation
800-532-5274
www.patientadvocate.org

Hospice Care

Hospice care helps to maintain quality of life and comfort towards the end of life. These organizations may point you to hospice programs in your area:

Caring Connections
800-658-8898
www.caringinfo.org

Family Caregiver Alliance (FCA)
800-445-8106
www.caregiver.org

National Family Caregivers Association (NFCA)
800-896-3650
www.nfcacares.org

Hospice Foundation of America
800-854-3402
www.hospicefoundation.org

National Hospice and Palliative Care Organization (NHPCO)
800-658-8898
www.nhpco.org

Palliative Care

Palliative care is care meant to provide the patient with pain relief, comfort, and a good quality of life. Good sources of information are as follows:

American Pain Foundation
888-615-PAIN (888-615-7246)
www.painfoundation.org

Cancer*Care*
800-813-HOPE (800-813-4673)
www.cancercare.org

Center to Advance Palliative Care
(212) 201-2670
www.capc.org

Support and Survivor Groups

Many patients and family members benefit from connecting with others who have dealt with the condition they are dealing with. In addition to the lung cancer–specific sites listed above, these resources may help:

Cancer Hope Network
877-HOPE-NET (877-467-3638)
www.cancerhopenetwork.org

Gilda's Club Worldwide
888-GILDA-4-U (888-445-3248)
www.gildasclub.org

LiveStrong Lance Armstrong Foundation

866-673-7205

www.livestrong.org

National Coalition for Cancer Survivorship (NCCS)

888-650-9127

www.canceradvocacy.org

Appendix C

Glossary

Activities of daily living (ADL): The normal actions taken each day, such as dressing, bathing, eating, and moving around

Acute: Having a sudden onset or arising very recently

Adenocarcinoma (ah deen oh KAR sih NOH muh): Cancer that begins in cells that line certain internal organs and have secretory properties, such as the cells lining the airways in lungs. These cells produce mucus.

Adjuvant therapy (ah-JOO-vant): Treatment given after the primary treatment to increase the chances of a cure. Adjuvant therapy for lung cancer may include chemotherapy and radiation therapy.

ADL: *See* activities of daily living.

Adrenal glands: Glands that sit on top of each kidney and produce hormones, such as adrenaline

Advanced cancer: Cancer that has spread beyond the original tumor to a distant part of the body

Agitation: A state of excess physical activity along with emotional distress, tension, or irritability

Alveoli (al VEE oh ly): The tiny air sacs in the lungs where oxygen and carbon dioxide are exchanged

Analgesic: A drug that relieves pain

Anemia: Too few red blood cells, a frequent side effect of chemotherapy

Anticonvulsant: A medication to prevent seizures

Antidepressant: A medication to relieve depression

Antiemetic: A medication to relieve nausea and vomiting

Anxiety: Sense of fear, concern, or uneasiness over an actual or anticipated problem

Aranesp: *See* darbepoetin.

Avastin: *See* bevacizumab.

Benign: A tumor that is not malignant or cancerous

Bevacizumab: A targeted therapy drug that blocks a tumor's ability to build blood vessels. The trade name is Avastin.

Biological therapy: A treatment that uses the body's own immune system to fight cancer or treatment side effects. Drugs to increase the production of red and white blood cells are often used as biological therapy.

Biopsy: The removal of a small amount of tissue, cells, or fluids from the body for examination under a microscope to detect cancerous cells

Brachytherapy: Radiation therapy using radioactive material sealed within a catheter and placed on or near the tumor for a brief period

Breakthrough pain: Increases in pain that occur despite the regular use of pain medication

Bronchi (BRONG ky): The airways in the lungs. The pleural of *bronchus*.

Bronchiole (BRONG kee ole): The tiniest airways in the lungs. Bronchioles end in alveoli, or air sacs.

Bronchoscope (BRON koh skope): A thin, tubular instrument with a light and videochip on the end that is inserted into the airways to examine them

Bronchoscopy (bron KOS koh pee): Using a bronchoscope to examine the airways of the lungs

Bronchus (BRONK us): An airway in the lung. The pleural is *bronchi*.

Cancer: Abnormal, uncontrolled cell growth; a malignant tumor that can invade local tissues and spread throughout the body

Carboplatin: A platinum-based drug used as first-line chemotherapy along with a second drug

Carcinoid: An uncommon lung tumor that grows and spreads more slowly than typical lung cancer

Carina (ka RYE na): The point where an airway branches into two airways

Central nervous system (CNS): The brain and spinal column

Cetuximab: A targeted therapy drug that works by binding to the epidermal growth factor receptors in cancer cells, thus blocking their activation. The trade name is Erbitux.

Chemotherapy: Drug treatment that kill rapidly growing cells, especially cancer cells, or keeps them from dividing and growing

Chest tube: A thin tube inserted into the chest after lung surgery to drain off fluids. Also used to drain fluid from a pleural effusion.

Chronic: An illness or condition that has a long duration

Cisplatin: A platinum-based drug used as first-line chemotherapy along with a second drug

Clinical trial: Research study involving people. Used to test ways of preventing, diagnosing, and treating illnesses. *See also* phase III trial.

CNS: *See* central nervous system.

Combination chemotherapy: Chemotherapy using two or more drugs

Comfort care: Care designed to keep the patient comfortable and pain-free with a good quality of life without attempting to cure the cancer. *See also* palliative care.

Complementary medicine: Noncurative therapies used alongside regular medical care to help patients feel better. Common complementary therapies include meditation and acupuncture.

Complete response: The disappearance of all signs of cancer in response to treatment. Also called complete remission.

Constipation: Bowel movements that are less frequent than usual and may be hard and difficult to pass

Colony stimulating factor drugs: *See* granulocyte colony-stimulating factors.

CT scan: An imaging process that creates a detailed sectional view of a part of the body

Cure: The remission of signs or symptoms of cancer or other disease for the remainder of one's life

Darbepoetin: A biological therapy that stimulates the bone marrow to produce more red blood cells. The trade name is Aranesp.

Deep vein thrombosis (DVT): A dangerous blood clot that forms in a vein deep inside the leg

Depression: A state of deep sadness characterized by inactivity, feelings of hopelessness, difficulty thinking and concentrating, marked changes in appetite and sleep patterns, and sometimes suicidal thoughts or actions.

Diaphragm: The dome-shaped breathing muscle in the abdomen that moves the lungs up and down during exhalation and inhalation

Disease progression: The worsening of a disease over time

DVT: *See* deep vein thrombosis.

Dyspnea (DISSP nee ah): Shortness of breath; painful or difficult breathing

Epoetin alfa (ee POH eh tin AL fuh): A biologic drug that stimulates the bone marrow to produce more red blood cells. Trade names are Epogen and Procrit.

Epogen: *See* epoetin alfa.

Esophagus: The tube that connects the mouth and throat to the stomach

Erbitux: *See* cetuximab.

Erlotinib (er LOH ty nib): Targeted therapy drug in a class of drugs called tyrosine kinase inhibitors. Kills cancer cells from the inside by interfering with the epidermal growth factor process. The trade name is Tarceva.

Etoposide: A drug commonly used along with a platinum-based drug as first-line chemotherapy for lung cancer

External beam radiation therapy: Radiation delivered from outside the body and aimed at the cancerous area

Extensive-stage small cell lung cancer: Small cell lung cancer that has spread outside the lung to other parts of the body, such as the liver, kidneys, or brain

Fatigue: Extreme, long-lasting tiredness, often a side effect of chemotherapy or radiation therapy

Filgrastim: A biologic drug used to stimulate the production of white blood cells. The trade name is Neupogen.

Fine-needle aspiration: A biopsy method that uses a needle inserted into the suspect area to remove a small sample of cells

Gamma knife: A type of external radiation equipment that delivers a very focused high-dose beam. *See* stereotactic radiosurgery.

G-CSF drugs: *See* granulocyte colony-stimulating factors.

Granulocyte colony-stimulating factors (G-CSFs): Drugs that help the body produce white blood cells. Used for treating neutropenia from chemotherapy.

Hemoptysis (he MOP ti sis): Coughing up blood

Hospice: Comprehensive palliative care for people who are terminally ill and no longer receiving treatment that is meant to be curative. Hospice care is sometimes at a residential facility but is most often provided at home by a specialized care team.

Hypercalcemia: Excess calcium in the blood

Intravenous (IV): Delivered through a vein

Laxative: A drug that is used to relieve constipation

Leukine: *See* sargramostim.

Limited-stage small cell lung cancer: Small cell lung cancer found only in one lung and nearby lymph nodes

Lobe: A section of the lung

Lobectomy: Surgical removal of a lobe of a lung

Localized cancer: Cancer that is confined to the original tumor and nearby tissues

Lung cancer: Cancer that forms in the tissues of the lungs, usually in the cells lining the air passages. The two main types are small cell lung cancer and non–small cell lung cancer.

Lung nodule: A relatively round lesion or area of abnormal tissue located within the lung

Lungs: Two spongy, saclike breathing organs in the chest that provide the body with oxygen and dispose of carbon dioxide

Lymph node: Small, bean-shaped structure that collects lymph, the clear fluid that bathes all the cells in the body and carries waste products away from the cells. Lymph nodes form chains in the body and are often the first place a cancer spreads to.

Malignant: Capable of invading tissues and spreading to other parts of the body. Another word for *cancerous*.

Mediastinoscope: A thin, tubular instrument with a light and lens on the end used to inspect the mediastinum. Tiny tools on the instrument can be used to collect biopsy samples.

Mediastinoscopy: Inserting a mediastinoscope into the chest area between the lungs to view the area and obtain biopsy samples

Mediastinum (media STY num): The space in the chest between the lungs

Metastases (meh TAS tuh seez): Tumors that are the result of the spread of a cancer from the cancer's original site

Metastasis (meh TAS tuh sis): Singular of *metastases*

Metastatic (meht a STAT ick): A cancer that has spread from its original site to another part of the body

Mucositis: Painful inflammation of the mouth and throat; a common side effect of chemotherapy

Narcotic: An opioid drug such as morphine or oxycodone. Principally used to control pain.

Nausea: Uneasy, unsettled feeling in the stomach along with an urge to vomit

Neulasta: *See* pegfilgrastim.

Neupogen: *See* filgrastim.

Neurologist: A doctor specializing in treating the brain and nerves

Neuropathy (noo ROP uh thee): *See* peripheral neuropathy.

Neutropenia: An abnormally low level of neutrophils, a type of white blood cell that helps prevent infection

Neutrophil: A type of white blood cell that is very important for preventing infection

Nonopioid: A pain medication, such as acetaminophen (Tylenol) or ibuprofen (Advil), that does not contain a narcotic drug

Non–small cell lung cancer (NSCLC): The most common type of lung cancer, characterized by abnormal cells that are larger than those in small cell lung cancer. *See also* adenocarcinoma and squamous cell carcinoma.

NSCLC: *See* non–small cell lung cancer.

Oncologist: A doctor who specializes in treating cancer

Oncology: The study of cancer, from the Greek word *oncos,* meaning mass or tumor

Opioid (OH pee OYD): A narcotic drug, such as morphine or oxycodone, used to treat moderate to severe pain

Oxygen therapy: Providing supplemental oxygen to help a patient breathe more easily

Pain management: Relieving cancer pain through drugs, injections, radiation, and other methods

Palliative (PA lee uh tiv) care: Care that is meant to relieve symptoms, provide comfort, and maintain quality of life but not to cure. *See also* comfort care.

Paraneoplastic syndrome: Signs and symptoms that occur because a cancer is producing an active substance or the body is reacting to the cancer at a distance from the tumor

Pathologist: A doctor who specializes in the diagnosis of disease by examining tissue under the microscope

PCI: *See* prophylactic cranial irradiation.

PDQ: Physician Data Query, a comprehensive database of cancer information maintained by the National Cancer Institute

Pegfilgrastim: A biologic drug used to stimulate the production of white blood cells in the bone marrow. The trade name is Neulasta.

Pericardial effusion: An accumulation of fluid in the sac surrounding the heart

Peripheral neuropathy (noo ROP un thee): Numbness, tingling, and pain in the feet and hands caused by some chemotherapy drugs

PET scan: An imaging study that uses radioactive glucose to detect tumors

Phase III trial: A study to compare the results of people taking a new treatment with results of people taking the standard treatment. The goal is to learn which group does better, for example by having fewer side effects or longer survival.

Placebo: A harmless, inactive substance given instead of a drug or other substance during a clinical trial

Platelets (thrombocytes): Tiny particles in the blood necessary for clotting

Pleura (PLOO uh): A thin tissue that covers the lungs and lines the inside of the chest to protect and cushion the lungs

Pleural cavity: The space between the layers of the membrane that lines the lungs and chest wall

Pleural effusion: An abnormal accumulation of fluid in the pleural cavity

Pleural fluid: Liquid found in the pleural cavity. Normal pleural fluid lubricates the layers and allows the lungs to move smoothly during respiration.

Pleurodesis: A technique used to close off the pleural cavity, usually by inducing scarring, to prevent pleural effusion

Pneumonectomy: Surgical removal of an entire lung

Pneumonia: An infection within the lung

Pneumonitis: General term for inflammation in the lung

Primary tumor: The main cancerous mass. Any spread of the cancer originates from the primary tumor.

Procrit: *See* epoetin alfa.

Prognosis: The likely course of the disease based on the usual progression and the individual characteristics of the patient

Progression-free survival: The time a cancer patient lives without any detectable increase or worsening of the disease

Prophylactic cranial irradiation (PCI): Radiation treatment of the brain to help prevent metastases to the brain

Pulmonary embolus: A blood clot in the lung

Pulmonologist: A doctor who specializes in treating lung problems

Quality of life: The ability to participate in and get satisfaction from the activities of daily living

Radiation oncologist: A doctor specializing in radiation therapy

Radiation therapy: Administering targeted, high-energy radiation to the affected area to kill cancer cells while avoiding healthy tissue

Radiosurgery: Using a very focused beam (or beams) of radiation to delivery very high energy doses in a highly targeted manner to the tumor to kill the cancer cells

Randomized clinical trial: A clinical trial in which patients are randomly assigned to receive standard therapy or a variation on standard therapy that includes the drug or other method that is under study

Recurrent cancer: Cancer that has returned after treatment

Resection: Surgical removal of part of an organ, such as removing a lobe of the lung

Respiratory system: The breathing organs, including the nose, mouth, trachea, lungs, and diaphragm

Respiratory therapist: A trained individual who specializes in helping patients use breathing medications and support devices

Respiratory therapy: Treatment for breathing problems, including supplemental oxygen

Risk factor: Anything, such as smoking or genetic heritage, that increases the likelihood of developing a particular health problem

Sargramostim: A biologic drug that stimulates the bone marrow to produce more white blood cells. The trade name is Leukine.

SCLC: *See* small cell lung cancer.

Screening: Routinely examining patients at risk for developing a certain health problem prior to developing symptoms or signs of the health problem

Sedative: A drug used to calm and relieve anxiety, agitation, depression, or insomnia

Seizure: Sudden, abnormal activity in the brain that causes a variety of symptoms, including brief loss of consciousness, lapses of awareness, sudden jerking of muscles, and convulsions

Side effect: An undesirable secondary effect, such as nausea or fatigue, of a drug or other treatment whose primary purpose is to treat disease

Sleeve lobectomy: A surgical technique for removing an upper lobe of the lung while preserving the remaining portions of the lung

Small cell lung cancer: A type of lung cancer characterized by cells that are small and rounded under the microscope

Sputum: Matter discharged by the air passages. Also called mucus.

Sputum cytology: Examining sputum to find cancerous cells

Squamous cell: A thin, flat cell that lines the air passages in the lungs and resembles the scales of a fish

Squamous cell carcinoma: A type of non–small cell lung cancer

Stage: The extent of a cancer within the body

Staging: Determining the extent of a cancer within the body

Standard therapy: Treatment that has been shown, through experience and clinical trials, to be the best available therapy

Stent: A small tube used to prop open an airway or blood vessel.

Sternum: The breastbone.

Stereotactic radiotherapy: *See* radiosurgery.

Stereotactic radiosurgery: *See* radiosurgery.

Stomatitis: Painful mouth sores, a possible side effect of chemotherapy

Superior vena cava syndrome (SVCS): Difficulty breathing, coughing, and swelling caused by a tumor pressing on the superior vena cava vein in the chest

Supportive care: Care that is designed to keep the patient comfortable, pain-free, and with a good quality of life. *See also* comfort care.

SVCS: *See* superior vena cava syndrome.

Tarceva: *See* erlotinib.

Targeted therapy: Cancer treatment using a drug such as erlotinib or bevacizumab to block the internal processes of cancer cells

Terminal disease: Cancer that has progressed to the point where it can no longer be treated and death is near

Thoracentesis (THOH ruh sen TEE sis): Inserting a needle between the ribs into the pleural cavity to remove fluid from a pleural effusion

Thoracic surgeon: A surgeon who specializes in the chest area

Thoracoscope (thoh RAY koh skope): A thin, tubular instrument with a light and lens on the end that can be inserted into the chest to view the area. Tiny tools on the instrument can be used to collect biopsy samples.

Thoracoscopy (THOR uh KOS koh pee): Using a thoracoscope to view inside the chest area and, often, to take biopsy samples

Thoracotomy (THOR un KAH toh mee): General term for an open surgery to the lung or chest

Thorax: The chest

Thrombocytes: Tiny particles in the blood necessary for clotting. *See also* platelets.

Thrombocytopenia: Abnormally low platelets in the blood. Can cause clotting problems.

Thrush: Fungal infection, often of the mouth and throat, that is sometimes a side effect of chemotherapy

Trachea: The tube through which air passes from the nose to the lungs; windpipe

Tube thoracostomy: Inserting a tube between the ribs into the chest to drain fluid from a pleural effusion

Tumor: An abnormal collection of cells. Can be benign or cancerous.

VATS: *See* video-assisted thorascopic surgery.

Video-assisted thorascopic surgery: Surgery to the lung using a miniature video camera and tools inserted between the ribs

Watchful waiting: Carefully observing a potential health problem, such as a lung nodule, without treating it to see if it changes or requires treatment

Wedge resection: The surgical removal of a small portion of the lung

Whole brain radiation: External beam radiation to the entire brain to treat brain metastases

X-ray: An image produced by electromagnetic radiation of a part of the body

Index

About the Author

Peter Mazzone, MD, MPH, FRCPC, FCCP, is on staff and is Director of Education at the Cleveland Clinic's Respiratory Institute. In addition, he is Program Director of the Pulmonary and Critical Care Fellowship Program, Director of the Lung Cancer Program for the Respiratory Institute, and Director of the Pulmonary Rehabilitation Program. Dr. Mazzone is board certified in internal medicine, pulmonary medicine, and critical care medicine. His treatment interests include lung nodules, lung cancer, and intensive care unit medicine. His research interests focus on breath analysis, lung cancer diagnostics, lung nodule analysis, lung physiology assessment, and lung cancer screening.

About Cleveland Clinic

Cleveland Clinic, located in Cleveland, Ohio, is a not-for-profit multispecialty academic medical center that integrates clinical and hospital care with research and education.

Cleveland Clinic was founded in 1921 by four renowned physicians with a vision of providing outstanding patient care based upon the principles of cooperation, compassion, and innovation. *U.S. News & World Report* consistently names Cleveland Clinic as one of the nation's best hospitals in its annual "America's Best Hospitals" survey. Approximately 1,800 full-time salaried physicians and researchers at Cleveland Clinic and Cleveland Clinic Florida represent more than 100 medical specialties and subspecialties. In 2007 there were 3.5 million outpatient visits to Cleveland Clinic and 50,455 hospital admissions. Patients came for treatment from every state and from more than 80 countries. Cleveland Clinic's website address is *www.clevelandclinic.org.*

2001641/0000KB1-P

LaVergne, TN USA
09 October 2010
200164LV00008B/1/P